T0140264

Multimedia Systems and Applications

Series editor

Borko Furht

More information about this series at: http://www.springer.com/series/6298

Amit Kumar Singh • Basant Kumar
Ghanshyam Singh • Anand Mohan
Editors

Medical Image Watermarking

Techniques and Applications

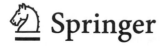 Springer

Editors
Amit Kumar Singh
Department of Computer Science
    and Engineering
Jaypee University of Information
    Technology
Waknaghat, Solan, Himachal Pradesh, India

Ghanshyam Singh
Department of Electronics and
    Communication Engineering
Jaypee University of Information
    Technology
Waknaghat, Solan, Himachal Pradesh, India

Basant Kumar
Department of Electronics and
    Communication Engineering
Motilal Nehru National Institute
    of Technology
Allahabad, Uttar Pradesh, India

Anand Mohan
Department of Electronics Engineering
Indian Institute of Technology (BHU)
Varanasi, Uttar Pradesh, India

Multimedia Systems and Applications
ISBN 978-3-319-86227-9   ISBN 978-3-319-57699-2   (eBook)
DOI 10.1007/978-3-319-57699-2

Printed on acid-free paper

This Springer imprint is published by Springer Nature
The registered company is Springer International Publishing AG
The registered company address is: Gewerbestrasse 11, 6330 Cham, Switzerland

Preface

Information and communication technology (ICT) has been potentially useful for cost-effective and speedy transmission of electronic patient record (EPR) over open channels for telemedicine applications. However, attempts of malicious attacks or hacking for unauthorized access, alteration, modification, deleting, or even preventing the transfer of EPR possess challenging tasks in the implementation of dependable telemedicine systems. Therefore, the authenticity of EPR and related medical images is of prime concern as they form the basis of inference for diagnostic purposes. In such applications, tamperproofing and guaranteed originality of EPR/medical images is achieved by embedding some kind of watermark(s) which must be secure and robust against malicious attacks. Although numerous robust watermarking algorithms have been proposed, there has been a rat race situation between the robustness of watermark and malicious attacks, making robust watermarking an interesting challenging area for researchers.

In view of addressing the above challenges of telemedicine systems concerned with the authenticity and security aspects of transmitted EPR/medical image(s) over open channels for telemedicine, this book presents the state-of-the-art medical image watermarking techniques and algorithms for telemedicine and other emerging applications. The book begins with a conceptual introduction of digital watermarking, important characteristics, novel applications, different watermarking attacks, and benchmark tools followed by a detailed literature review on spatial and transform domain medical image watermarking techniques, their merits, and limitations. Subsequently, an in-depth analysis of available techniques of medical image watermarking is highlighted with their limitations. Further, the book presents improved/novel methods of watermarking for e-health applications which offer higher robustness, better perceptual quality, increased embedding capacity, and a secure watermark. For telemedicine, tele-ophthalmology, telediagnosis, and tele-consultancy services, medical images play a prominent role for instant diagnosis and understanding of crucial diseases as well as to avoid the misdiagnosis. In order to overcome this problem, the book includes some improved/novel medical image watermarking methods. The book also explores the important spatial and transform domain techniques followed by the major performance matrices. Finally, the book includes emerging trends and research challenges in robust watermarking and watermark security with special reference to telemedicine applications.

The authors believe that the book would provide a sound platform for understanding the medical image watermarking paradigm and prove as a catalyst for researchers in the field and shall be equally beneficial for professionals. In addition, the book is also helpful for senior undergraduate and graduate students, researchers, and industry professionals working in the area as well as other emerging applications demanding robust watermarking.

The book contains ten chapters. Chapter 1 presents a brief introduction of digital watermarking techniques, their classification, important characteristics, and emerging applications of digital watermarks followed by the essential requirements of medical image watermarking.

Chapter 2 contains a detailed review of the literature on medical image watermarking techniques and algorithms using medical image(s) as covers because they offer higher data embedding capacity. It includes both, the computationally simple but fragile watermarking in "spatial domain" and computationally expensive "transform domain" techniques that offer robust watermarking. The spatial domain watermarking using least significant bit (LSB) substitutions and the correlation-based and spread-spectrum techniques are discussed wherein the watermark data is embedded directly by manipulating the pixel values, bit stream, or code values of the host signal (cover media). The transform domain watermarking modulates the coefficients of a transform, e.g., discrete Fourier transform (DFT), discrete cosine transform (DCT), discrete wavelet transform (DWT), and singular value decomposition (SVD). Computationally complex transform domain watermarking techniques offer superior robustness of watermarked data as compared to spatial domain techniques. The chapter specially focuses on wavelet-based watermarking because it offers major benefits of space-frequency localization, multi-resolution representation, multi-scale analysis, reducing blocking artifact, adaptability, and linear complexity besides being compatible with JPEG 2000 image coding.

Chapter 3 describes detailed techniques of watermarking in spatial and transform domains along with major performance evaluation parameters: peak signal-to-noise ratio (PSNR), weighted peak signal-to-noise ratio (WPSNR), mean square error (MSE), universal image quality index, structural similarity index measure (SSIM), normalized correlation (NC), noise visibility function (NVF), and bit error rate (BER) of the watermarking algorithms. In addition, this chapter also discusses important watermark attacks and the use of a standard benchmark tool to measure the robustness of watermarking algorithms.

Chapter 4 presents a new robust hybrid watermarking technique using fusion of DWT, DCT, and SVD instead of applying these techniques individually or in combination thereof. It is based on initially decomposing the host image into first-level DWT followed by transformation of low-frequency band (LL) and watermark image using DCT and SVD. Then, the singular vector of the watermark image is embedded in the singular component of the host image, and the watermarked image is generated by inverse SVD on modified singular vector and original orthonormal matrices, followed by inverse DCT and inverse DWT. The proposed method has been extensively tested and analyzed against known attacks such as JPEG, Gaussian, Salt-and-Pepper, Speckle, and Poisson. The experimental results have revealed that the proposed technique achieves superior performance in respect of imperceptibility, robustness, and capacity as compared to the techniques reported in literature. Watermark robustness has been checked using the benchmarking software "Checkmark," and it is found that the suggested algorithm is robust against the "Checkmark" attacks. Further, the performance of the proposed watermarking method by applying encryption on patient text data before embedding the watermark has been investigated.

Chapter 5 addresses the issue of faulty watermark due to channel noise distortions which may result into inappropriate disease diagnosis in telemedicine environment. The effect of channel noise distortions in creating faulty watermark has been minimized by encoding the watermark using error correction codes (ECCs) before embedding. The effects of Hamming, BCH, Reed–Solomon, and hybrid ECC consisting of BCH and repetition code on the robustness of text watermark and the cover image quality have been investigated. It is found that the hybrid ECC code has better performance as compared to that of the other three codes, and the suggested method is robust against known attacks without significant degradation of the cover image quality. Further, the performance of the proposed watermarking method by applying Reed–Solomon ECC on encrypted patient data before embedding the watermark has been presented. The robustness of this method has been checked using "Checkmark" and is found that the proposed method is robust against the "Checkmark" attacks.

Chapter 6 discusses the solution to the growing concern of medical identity theft. This is based on the development of new secure watermarking techniques of medical data/image using multiple watermarking where patient identity reference and telemedicine center logo are used as text watermark and image watermark, respectively, for identity authentication. The embedding of watermark is based on DWT and spread-spectrum where pseudorandom noise (PN) sequences are generated corresponding to each watermark bit of the image watermark. The spread-spectrum has been used to secure the image watermark, and enhancement in robustness of the text watermark has been achieved using BCH-based ECC before embedding. The performance of this watermarking method has been tested against known attacks. Subsequently, simultaneous embedding of three watermarks, i.e., doctor code, image reference code, and patient record using multilevel watermarking of cover medical image, has been proposed to address the issues of data security, data compaction, unauthorized access, and tamperproofing. The suggested method uses wavelet-based spread-spectrum watermarking where the encrypted text watermarks are embedded at multiple levels of the DWT sub-bands of the cover image. The performance of the developed scheme is evaluated and analyzed against known attacks by varying watermark sizes and the gain factor. It is reported that the suggested multilevel watermarking enhances the security of the patient data and thus it can be potentially useful in the prevention of patient identity theft.

In chapter 7, the authors proposed new secure multiple watermarking techniques using eye image as cover for secure and compact medical data transmission in tele-ophthalmology applications. The method is based on initially embedding of four different watermarks using fusion of DWT and SVD. A secure hash algorithm (SHA-512) is used for enhancing the security feature of the proposed watermarking technique. The performance in terms of "NC" and "BER" of the developed scheme is evaluated and analyzed against known signal processing attacks and "Checkmark" attacks. The method is found to be robust against all the considered attacks.

Chapter 8 contains an algorithm for multiple watermarking based on DWT, DCT, and SVD which can be extremely useful in the prevention of patient identity theft in medical applications. The proposed method uses three different watermarks in the form of medical lump image watermark, doctor signature, identification code, and diagnostic information of the patient as the text watermark for identity authentication purpose. In order to improve the robustness performance of the image watermark, back propagation neural network (BPNN) is applied to the extracted image watermark to reduce the noise effects on the watermarked image. The security of image watermark is also enhanced by using Arnold transform before embedding into the cover. Further, the symptom and signature text watermarks are also encoded by lossless arithmetic compression technique and Hamming error correction code, respectively. The compressed and encoded text watermark is then embedded into the cover image. The experimental results are examined by varying the gain factor, different sizes of text watermarks, and different cover image modalities. The results are provided to illustrate that the proposed method is able to withstand different signal processing attacks and has been found to give an excellent performance for robustness, imperceptibility, capacity, and security simultaneously. The robustness performance of the method is also compared with other reported techniques. Finally, the visual quality of the watermarked image is also evaluated by the subjective method. This shows that the visual quality of the watermarked images is acceptable for diagnosis at different gain factors.

In chapter 9, the authors presented a robust and secure multiple watermarking method using a combination of DWT, DCT, SVD, selective encryption, error correcting codes, and neural network. The proposed technique initially decomposes the host image into third-level DWT where the vertical frequency band at the second-level and low frequency sub-band at the third-level DWT are selected for embedding image and text watermark, respectively. Further, the proposed method addresses the issue of ownership identity authentication; multiple watermarks are embedded instead of a single watermark into the same multimedia objects simultaneously, which offer the extra level of security and reduced storage and bandwidth requirements in important applications areas. Moreover, the robustness image watermark is also enhanced by using "BPNN," which is applied on extracted watermark to minimize the distortion effects on the watermarked image. In addition, the method addresses the issue of channel noise distortions in identity information. This has been achieved using ECCs for encoding the text watermark before embedding into the host image. The effects of Hamming and BCH codes on the robustness of personal identity information in the form of text watermark and the cover image quality have been investigated. Recently, selective encryption is computationally fast for large size multimedia documents offering secure document dissemination for various multimedia applications. In order to reduce the computation time and enhance the security of the documents, selective encryption is applied on water-marked image, where only the important multimedia data is encrypted. The proposed method has been extensively tested and analyzed against known attacks. Based on experimental results, it is established that the proposed technique achieves superior performance in respect of robustness, security, and capacity with acceptable visual quality of the watermarked image as compared to reported techniques. Finally, we have evaluated the image quality of the watermarked image by subjective method.

Finally, chapter 10 discusses the recent trends and potential research challenges of the state-of-the-art watermarking techniques in brief. It includes medical image watermarking, 3D model watermarking, watermarking in cloud computing and multi-core environment, biometric watermarking, watermarking using mobile device, and securing online social network contents. The chapter also reviews several aspects about digital watermarking in different domains. Meanwhile, it discusses the requirements and potential challenges that the watermarking process faces.

This book is an extension of the Ph.D. thesis of Dr. Amit Kumar Singh submitted to the Department of Computer Engineering, National Institute of Technology (Institution of National Importance), Kurukshetra, Haryana, 2015, under the supervision of Dr. Mayank Dave and Prof. Anand Mohan.

First and foremost, the author is heartily thankful to *Prof. Borko Furht*, series editor, Multimedia Systems and Applications, for his guidance, promotion, encouragement, and support in every stage of my research work. His knowledge, kindness, patience, sincerity, and vision have provided me with lifetime benefits.

I am grateful to *Prof. S. P. Ghrera*, head of the Department of Computer Science & Engineering, Jaypee University of Information Technology, Waknaghat, Solan, Himachal Pradesh, for his consistent support, encouragement, and invaluable suggestions throughout the manuscript preparation. It is his enlightened guidance and vision and generous support that made it possible for me to finish this work within the stipulated time.

The authors are indebted to numerous colleagues for valuable suggestions during the entire period of the manuscript preparation.

We would also like to thank the publishers at Springer, in particular *Susan Lagerstrom-Fife*, senior publishing editor/CS Springer, for their helpful guidance and encouragement during the creation of this book.

We are sincerely thankful to all authors, editors, and publishers whose works have been cited directly/indirectly in this manuscript.

The authors would not justify their work without showing gratitude to their family members who have always been the source of strength to tirelessly work to accomplish the assignment. I owe my deepest gratitude toward my wife, *Sweta Singh*, for her continuous support and understanding of my goals and aspirations. Her infallible love and support has always been my strength. Her patience and sacrifice will remain my inspiration throughout my life. I am thankful to my daughters, *Anandi* and *Anaya*, for loving me and not complaining for their share of time I devoted for carrying out my work. I owe a lot to my parents, who encouraged and helped me at every stage of my personal and academic life and longed to see this achievement come true.

The second author, Dr. Basant Kumar, is also thankful to his wife, Dr. Namrata Parashar, and daughters, Anushka and Pragya, for sparing their time for this work. Further, the author wants to pay a deep sense of respect and gratitude to his grandfather (maternal) Sri Ram Uchit Singh for his life long support and his consistent encouragement and motivation for writing a book.

The third author, Prof. Ghanshyam Singh, is also thankful to his wife, Swati Singh; daughter, Jhanvi; and son, Shivam, for sparing their time for this work.

The fourth author, Prof. Anand Mohan, is also thankful to his wife, *Sudha Mohan*; daughter, *Amrita Mohan*; and son, *Ashish Mohan*, for their sparing time for this work.

Waknaghat, Solan, India   Amit Kumar Singh
Allahabad, India   Basant Kumar
Waknaghat, Solan, India   Ghanshyam Singh
Varanasi, India   Anand Mohan

Special Acknowledgments

We gratefully acknowledge the authorities of Jaypee University of Information Technology, Waknaghat, Solan, Himachal Pradesh, India, for their kind support to come up with this book.

Contents

List of Abbreviations

AES	Advanced Encryption Standard
ASCII	American Standard Code for Information Interchange
BCH	Bose, Chaudhuri, and Hocquenghem
BER	Bit error rate
CDMA	Code division multiple access
CS	Compressed sensing
DCT	Discrete cosine transform
DFT	Discrete Fourier transform
DIBR	Depth-image-based rendering
DICOM	Digital Imaging and Communications in Medicine
DWPT	Discrete wavelet packet transform
DWT	Discrete wavelet transform
ECC	Error-correcting codes
EPR	Electronic patient record
GA	Genetic algorithm
HMM	Hidden Markov model
HVS	Human visual system
ICA	Independent component analysis
ICT	Information and communication technology
IWT	Integer wavelet transform
LSB	Least significant bit
LZW	Lempel–Ziv–Welch
MPEG	The Moving Picture Experts Group
MSE	Mean square error
NC	Normalized correlation
NROI	Non-region of interest
NVF	Noise visibility function
PCA	Principal component analysis
PN	Pseudorandom noise
PSNR	Peak signal-to-noise ratio
QF	Quality factor

ROI	Region of interest
SNR	Signal-to-noise ratio
SPIHT	Set partitioning in hierarchical trees
SVD	Singular value decomposition
SVM	Support vector machine
WBCT	Wavelet-based contourlet transform

List of Figures

List of Tables

Chapter 1
Digital Image Watermarking: Concepts and Applications

Amit Kumar Singh, Basant Kumar, Ghanshyam Singh, and Anand Mohan

1.1 Introduction

In recent years, the digital document distribution over open channel using information and communication Technology (ICT) has proved an indispensible and cost effective technique for dissemination and distribution of digital media files. However, the prevention of copyright violation, ownership identification, and identity theft is still a challenging issue due to attempts of malicious attacks/hacking of open channel information. The prime motive behind this attacks/hacking is to alter, modify, or even cross-out the document watermark to illegally claim ownership or preventing the information transfer to intended recipients. Therefore, to address these critical challenges is an interesting problem for researchers in the field. The classic-model for invisible communication was first proposed by Simmons in 1984 as the prisoner's problem [1], which is shown in Fig. 1.1. The two prisoners in Fig. 1.1 want to develop an escape plan, but unfortunately all the communications between each other are arbitrated by warden.

A.K. Singh (✉)
Department of Computer Science & Engineering, Jaypee University of Information
Technology, Waknaghat, Solan, India
e-mail: amit_245singh@yahoo.com

B. Kumar
Department of Electronics and Communication Engineering, Motilal Nehru National
Institute of Technology, Allahabad, India
e-mail: singhbasant@yahoo.com

G. Singh
Department of Electronics and Communication Engineering, Jaypee University
of Information Technology, Waknaghat, Solan, India
e-mail: drghanshyam.singh@yahoo.com

A. Mohan
Department of Electronics Engineering, Indian Institute of Technology (BHU), Varanasi, India
e-mail: profanandmohan@gmail.com

© Springer International Publishing AG 2017
A.K. Singh et al. (eds.), *Medical Image Watermarking*, Multimedia Systems
and Applications, DOI 10.1007/978-3-319-57699-2_1

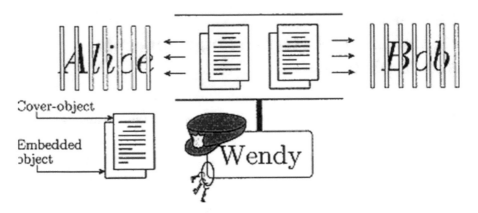

Fig. 1.1 The prisoner's problem [2]

They are not allowed to communicate through encryption and if any suspicious communication is noticed, the two prisoners will be placed in solitary confinement and thus preventing any exchange of information. Therefore, the prisoners must communicate invisibly in order not to arouse warden suspicion and they thought of hiding meaningful information in some cover message. To implement this, one of the prisoners created a picture of a blue cow lying on a green meadow and sent it to other prisoner. On this way, the Warden is unable to perceive the colours of objects in the picture that is transmitting some information, which is an example of data hiding. As an evident from the above example, the *data hiding* is a technique to hide data into a cover message without creating any perceptual distortion of the cover for identification, annotation and copyright. However, the constraints that affect the data hiding process [3] are: the quantity of data to be hidden, the need for invariance of these data under conditions where a cover (host) media is subjected to distortions like lossy compression, and degree to which the data must be immune to interception, modification, or removal by third party. Fundamentally, the data hiding techniques can be classified into two categories: (1) digital watermarking and (2) steganography [4]. The digital watermarking is a process of embedding data (called a watermark) into digital multimedia cover objects in such a way that the watermark can be detected or extracted later to make an assertion about the authenticity and/or originality of the object [5]. The basic concept of digital watermarking is closely related to the steganography (also known as covered writing) which emphases on bandwidth of the hidden message while concealing a message, image, or file within another message, image, or file, however in the case of watermarking, the watermark robustness is the key performance parameter.

The watermarking technique has been in use for several centuries however the field of digital watermarking and its wide applications have exponentially grown over the last 30 years due to modern developments in multimedia data processing, advancements in digital signal processing, and availability of high speed computational platforms. The watermarking is being potentially used for ownership assertion, fingerprinting, copy prevention/control, secure telemedicine, e-commerce, e-governance, media forensics, digital libraries, web publishing, media file archiving, artificial intelligence [6–8], and digital cinema [9] wherein a watermark can be embedded in every frame. In view of these interesting applications of watermarking, it has drawn focused attention in the present work and thus discussed in detail.

1.2   Importance and Necessity of Watermarking

Although, cryptography is the commonly used technique to protect digital content but it cannot provide facility to the owner to monitor as to how the content is handled after decryption. This limitation of cryptography may lead to illegal copying and distribution or misuse of the private information. The cryptographic techniques protect content in transit but after decryption of content it has no further protection. This major limitation of cryptography has been addressed in watermarking that protects the content even after decryption. Watermarking techniques embed imperceptible watermarking information into the main content such that the watermark is neither removed during normal usage nor causes inconvenience to the users. A watermark can be designed to survive different processes such as decryption, re-encryption, compression and geometrical manipulations [10]. In recent times, telemedicine applications have started playing important role in the development and use of technology in the medical field. Digital imaging and communications in medicine (DICOM) is a basic criterion to communicate electronic patient record (EPR) data. In DICOM, a header containing important information about the patient is also attached with the medical image file. Protection of this header during transmission, and storage is an important issue which can be effectively addressed by watermarking to achieve guarantied security and authenticity [11].

1.3   Classifications of Digital Watermarks

Figure 1.2 shows general classification of the watermarking techniques [5]. Depending upon the type of data to be watermarked, the watermarking methods can be classified into four categories: text watermarking, image watermarking, audio watermarking, and video watermarking. However, due to higher data embedding capacity of image, the present work focuses on watermarking using image as cover media. According to the human perception, the watermarks can be divided into three different types: visible watermark, Invisible-Robust watermark, Invisible-Fragile watermark and Dual watermark. Visible watermark is a secondary translucent overlaid into the primary image. The watermark appears visible to a casual viewer on a careful inspection. The invisible-robust watermark is embedded in such a way that alterations made to the pixel values are perceptually not noticeable and the watermark can be recovered only with appropriate decoding mechanism. The invisible-fragile watermark is embedded in such a way that any manipulation or

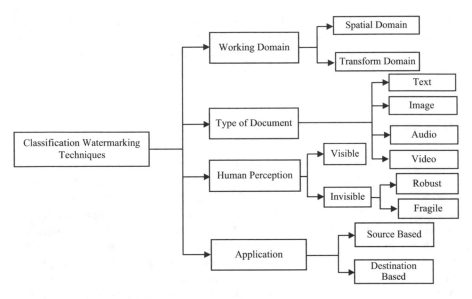

Fig. 1.2 Classification of watermarking techniques [5]

modification of the cover would alter or destroy the watermark. Dual watermark is a combination of a visible and an invisible watermark [5]. In this type of watermark an invisible watermark is used as a backup for the visible watermark. According to working domain, the watermark could be applied in spatial and transform domain.

From the application view point, the watermark could be *source* or *destination* based where the former is preferred for ownership identification or authentication and the latter is used for uniquely identifying the buyer. In source based watermarking a unique watermark identifying the owner is embedded in all the copies of the cover image being distributed whereas in destination based watermarking, each distributed copy gets a unique watermark identifying the particular buyer and it is used to trace the buyer in the case of illegal distribution/reselling. The watermarking techniques can also be classified into *reversible* and *irreversible* techniques [12, 13]. Reversible watermarking avoids irreversible distortions in the host cover image by using techniques that provide extraction of the watermark from the watermarked cover document. Therefore these techniques are preferred for medical image watermarking to reduce the probability of incorrect diagnosis.

1.4 Potential Characteristics of Digital Watermarks

The key characteristics of digital watermarks [14, 15] are:

1. Robustness: A digital watermark is called robust if it resists a designated class of transformations and thus can be used for copyright protection. The robustness criterion focuses on two issues i.e. (1) whether or not the watermark is present after distortion in the data and, (2) whether it can be detected by the watermark detector.

2. Imperceptibility: The imperceptibility can be considered as a measure of perceptual transparency of watermark and it refers to the similarity of original and watermarked images.
3. Capacity: It is the amount of information that can be embedded in a cover. This amount of information highly depends on the applications such as copyright protection, fingerprinting, authentication and confidentiality of medical data, as the information to be embedded may be a logo image, a number etc.
4. Security: The security of watermark implies that the watermark should be difficult to remove or alter without damaging the cover image. The level of watermark security requirement can vary depending upon the application.
5. Data-payload: The data payload of a watermark can be defined as the amount of information that it contains e.g. if a watermark contains 'n' bits, then there are 2^n possible watermarks with actually 2^{n+1} possibilities as one possibility can be that no watermark is present. A good watermark should contain all the required data within any arbitrary and small portion of the cover.
6. Fragility: The fragile watermark basically aims at the content authentication. This is reverse of the robustness criterion. The watermarks may be designed to withstand various degrees of acceptable modifications in the watermarks on account of distortions in the media content. Here, watermark differs from a digital signature which requires 100% match.
7. Computational cost: The computational cost basically refers to the cost of embedding the watermark into a cover and extracting it from the digital cover. In some applications, it is important that the embedding process be as fast and simple as possible while the extraction can be more time consuming. In other applications, the speed of extraction is absolutely crucial.
8. Tamper resistance: Tamper-detection of watermarks is used to check the authenticity of digital photographs. Watermarks of this type are sensitive to any change of the watermark data; thus, by checking the integrity of the watermark, the system can determine whether or not the watermark has ever been modified or replaced.

1.5   Framework for Watermarking

In general, the watermarking system consists of two processes - encoding and extraction process [4] as shown in Fig. 1.3. Referring Fig. 1.3a it is evident that there are three inputs: a watermark, the original cover media and the optional public or secret key to generate a watermarked image. Figure 1.3a depicts the extraction process which takes the input as watermarked image/original data (cover), secret or public key and test data from which cover image and its proprietorship can be determined [16, 17].

Therefore from Fig. 1.3a, a general watermarked cover image (W) is expressed as the function (F) of watermark data (W_d), a cover data (C_d) and a secret key (K) i.e.

$$W = F\left(W_d, C_d, K\right) \qquad (1.1)$$

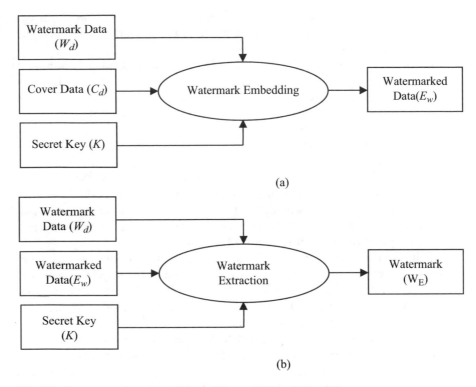

Fig. 1.3 The watermark process (**a**) embedding and (**b**) extraction [4]

The watermark embedding process is defined as:

$$\text{Watermark Embedding}\left(E_w\right) = F\left(W_d, C_d, K\right) \tag{1.2}$$

Further, the watermark extraction process is defined as:

$$\text{Watermark Extraction}\left(W_E\right) = F\left(W \, or \, C_d, E_w, K\right) \tag{1.3}$$

1.6   Recent Applications of Digital Watermark

A main application of the digital watermark is depicted in Fig. 1.4. The important and latest potential applications are [7, 8, 15, 18] as follows.

1. *Fingerprinting*: It is the mechanism in which the watermarked content contains the intended recipient's identification information in order to trace back the source of illegal distribution.

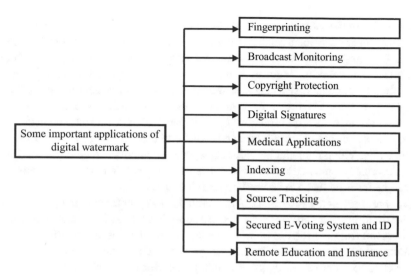

Fig. 1.4 Potential applications of watermarking

2. *Broadcast monitoring*: The broadcast monitoring is an application which enables content owners to automatically verify where, when and how long their content was broadcast via terrestrial, cable or satellite television. Also, the e-commerce has become a huge business and a driving factor in the development of the Internet. Online shopping services and online delivery of digital media, is very popular today and will become an increasingly important part of e-commerce and mobile e-commerce. The digital watermarking techniques play an important role to protect an intellectual property in e-governance, e-commerce applications, copy control, media identification and tracking.

3. *Copyright protection*: Providing copyright protection to digital data by hiding secret information is main goal of digital watermarking. Many content owners to embed digital watermarks in images as a means to communicate and protect image copyrights. This ensures that image users or licensees are acting in compliance with guidelines and allows legal departments to effectively communicate and enforce image copyrights.

4. *Digital signatures*: A mechanism employed in public-key cryptosystems that enables the originator of an information object to generate a signature, by encipherment (using a private key) of a compressed string derived from the object. The digital signature can provide a recipient with proof of the authenticity of the object's originator.

5. *Medical applications*: In this application the watermarking provides both authentication and confidentiality in a reversible manner without affecting the medical image in any way. Recently, telemedicine, tele-ophthalmology, tele-diagnosis, tele-consultancy, tele-cardiology, tele-radiology applications play an important role in the development of the medical field. However, protect the transmission, storage and sharing of EPR data between two hospitals or via open/unsecured

channel are the most important issues in this field. Telemedicine can be divided into number of medical related technologies using computers for health care like tele-radiology, tele-pathy, tele-care, telesurgery, tele-neurology etc. Medical image watermarking requires extreme care when embedding additional data within the medical images because the additional information must not affect the image quality. Confidentiality, authentication, integrity and availability are important security requirements with EPR data exchange through open channels. All these security requirements can be fulfilled using suitable watermarks.

6. *Indexing*: Video mail can be indexed, where comments can be embedded in the video content; movies and news items can also be, where markers and comments can be inserted that can be used by search engine.

7. *Source tracking*: A watermark is embedded into a digital signal at each point of distribution. If a copy of the work is found later, then the watermark may be retrieved from the copy and the source of the distribution is known.

8. *Secured e-voting systems*: With rapid growth of computer network, Internet has reached to common villagers of country and worldwide as well. Due to widespread use of the Internet with information and communication technologies in order to get their inevitable benefits like accuracy, speed, cost saving etc. more secure transactions such as shopping, banking, submitting tax returns are done online. Obviously, electronic voting is a possible alternative for conducting elections by maintaining security in election process. For the election commission of India and other countries to conduct free and fair polls is always be challenging task. Current research focuses on designing and building 'voting protocols' that can support the voting process, while implementing the security mechanisms required for preventing fraud and protecting voters' privacy. So we need a highly secured e-voting system is required. Further, digital watermarks are also used to protect state driver licenses by providing covert and machine readable layer of security to fight against various issues such as digital counterfeiting, fraud, identity theft etc. [19].

9. *Remote education and insurance companies*: Due to the shortage of teachers and other problems in rural areas in, distance education is gaining popularity of developing any diverse countries. So there is a strong need for intelligent technologies to create a deployable remote education solution. However, dissemination of valuable content and teacher-student interaction are some of the major challenges in the distance education solution. The secured transmission of data is part of distant learning. Digital watermarking may provide one of the important solutions for the remote education. Also, different insurance companies such as health and vehicle nowadays use image processing application. Health insurance companies are storing the scanned copies of the medical data of their clients. The database may require processing and transmitting to central administrative offices. The car companies' image databases are referred for insurance-related decision making in case of damage to vehicles during accidents. The digital image watermarking protection is provided to such image database.

1.7   Essential Requirements for Medical Image Watermarking

In recent time, tele-medicine, tele-ophthalmology, tele-diagnosis and tele-consultancy services, medical images play a prominent role for instant diagnosis, understanding of crucial diseases as well as to avoid the misdiagnosis. Further, medical identity theft has been a serious security concern in telemedicine [20, 21]. Robert Siciliano, CEO of IDTheftSecurity.com, an identity theft expert, says, that would be a big fat yes. It's almost like the perfect crime as far as medical identity theft is concerned. The long-distance nature of this type of treatment fuels the anonymity of it all [22]. Medical images contain sensitive information, and when they are transmitted over the unsecured network, they become vulnerable to corruption by noisy transmission channels and attacks by hackers or individuals with malicious intents. These attacks may include obtaining confidential information about the patient, changing patient information in the image header, and tampering with the image pixel content. In addition to that medical identity theft is a growing and dangerous crime and identity theft resource center produced a survey shown that the medical-related identity theft accounted for nearly half of all identity thefts as reported in the United States in 2013, *USA Today* reports said [23]. These demand development of secure medical data/image watermarking schemes. Figure 1.5 shows the some potential advantages of medical image watermarking. The major advantages of the medical image watermarking [24–27] are:

1. Smaller storage space is required for storing the medical image and the patient record together as the patient record is embedded inside the image.
2. Reduced bandwidth requirement during transmission as the additional requirement of bandwidth for the transmission of the metadata can be avoided if the data is hidden in the image itself.

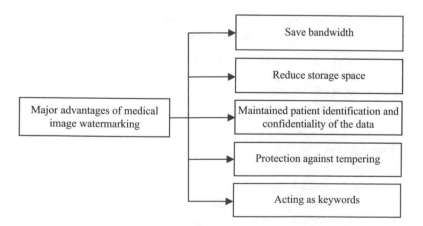

Fig. 1.5 Main advantages of medical image watermarking

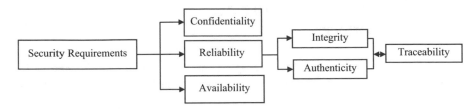

Fig. 1.6 Major security requirements for EPR data [29]

3. Ownership identification and confidentiality of the patient data is maintained as this data is hidden in the cover image.
4. Protection against tampering as the after-effects of a tampered medical data may cost a life due to wrong diagnosis.
5. The hidden watermarks can play the role of keywords, based on which efficient archiving and data retrieval from querying mechanisms take place. Further, it provides a valuable solution for potential issues such as medical data management and distribution [28].

However, the medical image watermarking requires extreme care when embedding additional data within the medical images because the additional information must not affect the image quality. The electronic patient record (EPR) data exchange through unsecured channels required high degree of security. As depicted in Fig. 1.6, it includes three mandatory security requirements [29]:

1. Confidentiality means only the authorized users have to access the information.
2. Reliability has two important outcomes: (a) Integrity—the information has not been modified by unauthorized people, and (b) Authentication—a proof that the information belongs indeed to the correct source. Further, the traceability is important components of the reliability and use to trace the information along its distribution.
3. The availability is an ability of information system to be used by entitled users in the normal scheduled conditions of access and exercise.

The authentication, integration and confidentiality are the most important issues concerned with EPR data exchange through unsecured channels [24, 29]. All these requirements can be fulfilled using suitable watermarks.

1.8 Summary

This chapter presented a brief introduction of digital watermarking, classification, important characteristics and recent applications of digital watermarks followed by the essential requirements of medical image watermarking. It has been observed that transmission, sharing and storage of electronic patient record (EPR) data through unsecured channels required high degree of security which includes confidentiality, reliability and availability in medical applications. The development of secure medical data/image watermarking is essential requirements in the area of medical fields which provide smaller storage space, reduced bandwidth requirement, ownership identification, confidentiality and protection against tampering for EPR data.

References

1. G.J. Simmons, The prisoners problem and the subliminal channel, in *Advances in Cryptology*, Proceedings of CRYPTO 83, (Plenum Press, New York, 1984), pp. 51–67
2. S. Craver, On public-key steganography, The presence of an active warden technical report RC 20931, IBM, 1997
3. W. Bender, D. Gruhl, N. Morimoto, A. Lou, Techniques for data hiding. IBM Syst. J. **35**(3&4), 313–336 (1996)
4. S. Katzenbeisser, F.A.P. Petitcolas, *Information hiding techniques for steganography and digital watermarking* (Artech House, London, 2000)
5. S.P. Mohanty, Watermarking of digital images, M.S. Thesis, Indian Institute of Science, India, 1999
6. N. Morimoto, Digital watermarking technology with practical applications. Inf. Sci. Special Issue on Multimedia Inf. Technol., Part 1 **2**(4), 107–111 (1999)
7. F. Hartung, F. Ramme, Digital rights management and watermarking of multimedia content for m-commerce applications. IEEE Commun. Mag. **38**((11), 78–84 (2000)
8. B.L. Gunjal, S.N. Mali, Applications of digital image watermarking in industries, pp. 5–7, CSI Communications, 2012
9. R. Chandramouli, N. Memon, M. Rabbani, Digital watermarking, encyclopedia of imaging. Sci. Technol., 1–21 (2002)
10. B.M. Irany, A high capacity reversible multiple watermarking scheme – applications to images, medical data, and biometrics, Master Thesis, Department of Electrical and Computer Engineering University of Toronto, 2011
11. S.A.K. Mostafa, N. El-sheimy, A.S. Tolba, F.M. Abdelkader, H.M. Elhindy, Wavelet packets-based blind watermarking for medical image management. Open Biomed. Eng. J. **4**, 93–98 (2010)
12. J.B. Feng, I.C. Lin, C.S. Tsai, Y.P. Chu, Reversible watermarking: current and key issues. Int. J. Network Security **2**(3), 161–170 (2006)
13. S. Lee, C.D. Chang, T. Kalker, Reversible image watermarking based on integer-to-integer wavelet transform. IEEE Trans. Inf. Foren. Security **2**(3), 330–321 (2007)
14. H.C. Huang, W.C. Fang, Techniques and application of intelligent multimedia data hiding. Telecommun. Syst. **44**(3-4), 241–251 (2010)
15. A.K. Singh, B. Kumar, M. Dave, S.P. Ghrera, A. Mohan, Digital image watermarking: techniques and emerging applications, handbook of research on modern cryptographic solutions for computer and cyber security, IGI Global, USA, pp. 246–272, 2016
16. F. Cayre, C. Fontaine and T. Furon, Watermarking security: theory and practice, IEEE Trans. Signal Process., 53 (10), 3976–3987 (2005)
17. L.P. Freire, P. Comesana, J.R. Troncoso-Pastoriza, F. Perez-Gonzalez, Watermarking security: a survey, in *Transactions on Data Hiding and Multimedia Security*, ed. by Y. Q. Shi (Ed), vol. 4300, (LNCS Springer, Berlin, 2006), pp. 41–72
18. A.K. Singh, M. Dave, A. Mohan, Wavelet based image watermarking: futuristic concepts in information security. Proc. Natl. Acad. Sci., India Sect. A: Phys. Sci. **84**(3), 345–359 (2014)
19. http://www.digitalwatermarkingalliance.org/faqs.asp

20. M. Terry, Medical identity theft and telemedicine security. Telemed. e-Health **15**(10), 928–932 (2009)
21. A.K. Singh, B. Kumar, M. Dave, A. Mohan, Multiple watermarking on medical images using selective DWT coefficients. J. Med. Imaging Health Inf. **5**(3), 607–614 (2015)
22. D. Bowman., http://www.fiercehealthit.com/story/researchers-use-digitalwatermarks-protect-medical-images (2012)
23. M. Ollove., www.usatoday.com/story/___/stateline-identity-thefts-medical___/5279351 (2014)
24. A.K. Singh, M. Dave, A. Mohan, Robust and secure multiple watermarking in wavelet domain, a special issue on advanced signal processing technologies and systems for healthcare applications (ASPTSHA). J. Med. Imaging Health Inf. **5**(2), 406–414 (2015)
25. A.K. Singh, B. Kumar, M. Dave, A. Mohan, Robust and imperceptible dual watermarking for telemedicine applications. Wirel. Pers. Commun. **80**(4), 1415–1433 (2014)
26. A. Sharma, A.K. Singh, S.P. Ghrera, Robust and secure multiple watermarking technique for medical images. Wirel. Pers. Commun. **92**(4), 1611–1624 (2017)
27. A.K. Singh, M. Dave, A. Mohan, Hybrid technique for robust and imperceptible multiple watermarking using medical images. J. Multimedia Tools Appl. **75**(14), 8381–8401 (2015)
28. A. Giakoumaki, S. Pavlopoulos, D. Koutsouris, Senior member, ieeemultiple image watermarking applied to health information management. IEEE Trans. Inf. Technol. Biomed. **10**(4), 722–732 (2006)
29. G. Coatrieux, H. Maitre, B. Sankur, Y. Rolland, R. Collorec, Relevance of watermarking in medical imaging, in Proceedings of the IEEE EMBS Conference on Information Technology Applications in Biomedicine, Arlington, USA, pp. 250–255, 2000

Chapter 2
Medical Image Watermarking Techniques: A Technical Survey and Potential Challenges

Amit Kumar Singh, Basant Kumar, Ghanshyam Singh, and Anand Mohan

2.1 Introduction

Recent advancements in high-bandwidth digital communication technologies has opened up newer opportunities of transmitting medical data across geographical boundaries through Internet, mobile networks, and other wireless/wired communication channels and thus covering rural/remote areas, accident sites, ambulance, and hospitals [1]. The transmission of medical data over an open communication channel poses different possibilities of threat that severely affect its authenticity, integrity, and confidentiality which demands for implementing some kind of medical watermarking scheme to avoid prompting attention and preventing access by an unintended recipient. The medical image watermarking provides a convenient platform to address these issues [2–6]. Despite the broad literature on various application fields, a very few work has been implemented towards the exploitation of health-oriented perspectives of watermarking [3, 5, 7–9]. The watermarking techniques in the area of

A.K. Singh (✉)
Department of Computer Science & Engineering, Jaypee University of Information Technology, Waknaghat, Solan, India
e-mail: amit_245singh@yahoo.com

B. Kumar
Department of Electronics and Communication Engineering, Motilal Nehru National Institute of Technology, Allahabad, India
e-mail: singhbasant@yahoo.com

G. Singh
Department of Electronics and Communication Engineering, Jaypee University of Information Technology, Waknaghat, Solan, India
e-mail: drghanshyam.singh@yahoo.com

A. Mohan
Department of Electronics Engineering, Indian Institute of Technology (BHU), Varanasi, India
e-mail: profanandmohan@gmail.com

© Springer International Publishing AG 2017
A.K. Singh et al. (eds.), *Medical Image Watermarking*, Multimedia Systems and Applications, DOI 10.1007/978-3-319-57699-2_2

telemedicine require extreme care when embedding additional data within the medical images because the additional information must not affect the image quality. The confidentiality, reliability and availability are important security requirements with electronic patient record (EPR) data exchange through unsecured channels [1, 5, 10].

The subsequent section of the chapter is structured as follows: Section 2.2 presents a brief literature review of current state-of-the-art medical as well as digital image watermarking techniques. Section 2.3 presents the potential challenges and fruitful discussion in the medical image watermarking techniques. Section 2.4 provides summary of the chapter.

2.2 Review of Available Watermarking Techniques

In this section, the authors are presenting a detailed literature review on the current state-of-the-art medical as well as digital image watermarking techniques using error correcting codes (ECC) [1, 2, 9, 11, 12], multiple watermarking methods [8, 13–15], hybrid techniques [16–44], watermarking using machine learning techniques [45–70], biometric watermarking [71, 72], watermarking with compression techniques [73–79] and some other perspectives of the watermrking [80–103]. Further, the techniques have been carried out to explore the limitations of existing techniques with special reference to their suitability in medical image watermarking. Some novel/improved state-of-the-art techniques are discussed below:

2.2.1 Watermarking Techniques Using Error Correcting Codes

In order to that Singh et al. [1, 12], Mostafa et al. [2], Giakoumaki et al. [9] and Terzija et al. [11] have proposed state-of-the-art technique to embed an encoded watermark with the help of error correcting codes (ECC) to improve the robustness of watermark. The ECC based watermarking methods attempt to find a trade-off between the number of bits to be embedded and the number of bit-errors that can be corrected. Singh et al. [1] proposed a medical image watermarking technique in which the technique embeds medical text watermarks into selected sub-band of discrete wavelet transform (DWT) cover medical image coefficients using spread-spectrum technique. In the embedding process, the cover image is decomposed up to third level DWT coefficients. Three different text watermarks are embedded into the selected horizontal and vertical sub-band DWT coefficients of the first, second and third level, respectively. The selection of these coefficients for embedding purpose is based on threshold criteria. Robustness of the proposed watermarking scheme is further enhanced by applying error correcting code to the ASCII representation of the text watermark and the encoded text watermark is finally embedded into the cover medical image. It is observed that the proposed scheme correctly extracts the embedded watermarks without error and provides high degree robustness against numerous known attacks while maintaining the imperceptibility of watermarked image. Mostafa et al. [2] have proposed a watermarking method for telemedicine applications, which provides a way to secure EPR information in order to reduce the storage space and transmission cost. In this method, the EPR information is embedded after the second level of decomposition of the cover image using discrete wavelet packet transform (DWPT). Here, the EPR information is initially coded using Bose, Ray-Chaudhuri, Hocquenghem (BCH) code and then embedded to improve the robustness. However, this method has the disadvantage of higher decoding time of BCH codes. Giakoumaki et al. [9] proposed a wavelet based multiple watermarking scheme for medical image. According to characteristic and requirements, different watermarks such as signature, index, caption and reference are assigned at different decomposition level and sub-bands of DWT coefficients of medical image and BCH error correcting codes are used to improve the robustness of the watermark.

Terzija et al. [11] proposed a method for improving efficiency and robustness performance of the watermarks by using three different error correction codes, namely, (15,7)-BCH, (7,4)-Hamming Code and (15-7)-Reed-Solomon code are investigated. These codes are applied to the ASCII representation of the text which is used as watermark. The watermark is embedded into the original cover image by first decomposing the cover up to second level using discrete DWT with the pyramidal structure and then the watermark is added to the largest DWT coefficients that represent high- and middle-frequencies of the cover image. It is shown that Reed-Solomon code performs better due to its excellent ability to correct errors, however, the ECCs considered are not able to deal with bit error rates (BER) greater than 10–20%. Singh et al. [12] also presents an ECCs based watermarking method in DWT-SVD domain using four different error correcting codes such as Hamming, the BCH, the Reed–Solomon and hybrid error correcting (BCH and repetition code) codes for encoding of text watermark in order to achieve additional robustness for sensitive text watermark. The performance of proposed algorithm is evaluated against various signal processing attacks by varying the strength of watermarking and covers image modalities. The experimental results demonstrate that this algorithm provides better robustness without affecting the quality of watermarked image. Among the four error correcting codes tested, it has been observed that the hybrid code achieves better results in terms of robustness.

2.2.2   Multiple Watermarking Techniques

For the ownership identity authentication purpose, multiple watermarking methods have been proposed by Giakoumaki et al. [8], Navas et al. [13], Kannammal et al. [14], Singh et al. [15] to achieve higher security than single watermarks. Giakoumaki et al. [8] described wavelet-based multiple watermarking scheme that addresses the problems of medical confidentiality protection. This method uses third level decomposition of the cover image using DWT to embed the watermarks into selected detailed coefficient of cover image. To extract multiple watermark bits, a quantization function is applied to each of the marked coefficients. The advantages of this method are its robustness, reliability, efficiency, reduced distortion and resistance to attacks. However, it involves higher computational complexity. Navas et al. [13] have proposed a blind method for telemedicine applications based on integer wavelet transform (IWT) which groups the wavelet coefficients of the cover image into different wavelet blocks based on human visual system (HVS). The EPR data is first encrypted and then embedded into the non-Region of Interest (NROI) part of the cover medical image. Region of Interest (ROI) part containing the important medical information for diagnosis is stored without any noise. The proposed method can embed and recover at most '3400' characters without any noise that is important for EPR information hiding but the computational cost of this method is high.

Kannammal et al. [14] proposed a digital watermarking method where ECG and patients' demographic text act as two level watermarks. During embedding, DWT is applied on the original image and the image is decomposed into three sub-bands. Next, the texture matrix for each sub-band is calculated. The wavelet coefiicients are selected for watermarking using threshold values. The method can be used for providing authentication, confidentiality and integrity of the medical information. Singh et al. [15] proposed a wavelet based spread-spectrum multiple watermarking scheme considering medical watermarks in the form of both text and image. The experimental results are obtained by varying the watermark size and gain factor. The performance of developed scheme has been evaluated against various attacks. The robustness of text watermark has been enhanced by using BCH code.

2.2.3 Hybrid Watermarking Techniques

Further, some noted researchers are using *hybrid watermarking* techniques to enhance the performance of watermarking systems [16–44]. Lou and Sung [16] described two transform methods (DCT and DWT) to embed a random watermark into an image. After the third level decomposition of the cover image by DWT, DCT is applied to the selected sub-bands (HL3 and LH3). These DCT coefficients are recorded in zig-zag order. A watermark of zero means and variance of one is embedded into these sub-bands. The original image is not required for watermark extraction process. The experimental results show that the proposed method keeps the image quality good and robust against known attacks. Ouhsain et al. [17] have proposed a watermarking method using multiple parameters discrete fractional Fourier (MPDFRF) and DWT. In this embedding process, the cover image is decomposed into four wavelet sub-bands using DWT. After each sub-band is segmented into blocks, the MPDFRF transform is applied to each block. The watermark image is then embedded into the blocks. The experimental results show the good visual imperceptibility and robustness against known attacks. Jiansheng et al. [18] have proposed an algorithm for digital image watermarking based on DWT and DCT. This method of embedding uses decomposition of the host image into multilevel (n = 3) wavelet transform and the DCT coefficients of the watermark is embedded in the high frequency band of DWT coefficients. In this method, the high frequency coefficients are plotted into 2 × 2 image sub blocks, and entropy and square values of each image sub-block is calculated. The experimental result shows that the method is robust against known signal processing attacks.

Hadi et al. [19] proposed a method based on two transform methods, Fresnel and DWT. Before embedding the watermark, the cover image is transformed first by Fresnel transform to generate the encrypted cover image. After the second decomposition of cover image using DWT, the encrypted copyright information is embedded into the decomposed cover image. The method uses chaotic sequence as key to encrypt the copyright information. The chaotic sequence is very sensitive to any change in its value, so that the eavesdropper has to obtain exactly its value which is difficult and time consuming. However, encrypting the copyright information before watermarking has become unavoidable, but the delay encountered during embedding and extraction of the watermark is also an important factor in telemedicine applications. Cao et al. [20] proposed an adaptive blind watermarking method based on DWT and Fresnel diffraction transform. Initially, the cover image is decomposed (up to third level) by DWT, the binary kinoform of the watermark image is embedded. The experimental results have shown that the watermark image via Fresnel diffraction transforms has good concealment performance. The kinoform is more secure than simple permutation. However, the proposed method is suitable for binary digital watermark only. Lai and Tsai [21] proposed a hybrid image-watermarking scheme based on DWT and SVD. The method applied SVD on the selected sub-band of the DWT cover image and the singular values of the selected sub-bands of the cover image are modified with half of the watermark image. The watermark extraction is just reversing the embedding process. With SVD, small modification of singular values does not affect the visual recognition of the cover image, which improves the robustness and transparency of the method. However, both the computational cost and storage space requirements in this method are high. Nakhaie and Shokouhi [22] have proposed a no-reference objective quality measurement method based on spread-spectrum technique and DWT using ROI processing. In this embedding process, the original image is first divided into two separate parts, ROI and NROI, and DWT and DCT are applied on ROI and NROI parts, respectively. The binary watermark is embedded into DCT transform of NROI part of the cover image.

Ahire and Kshirsagar [23] proposed a blind watermarking algorithm based on DCT-DWT that embeds a binary image into the gray image. After the third level decomposition by DWT, the selected sub-bands are divided into block of 4 × 4. The DCT is applied on each block. For embedding binary watermark information corresponding pseudorandom sequences are added in the middle frequency coefficients of the DCT block. The watermark extraction process is same as the embedding process but in reverse order. Its advantages are that the proposed algorithm takes the full advantages of the multi resolution and energy compression of DWT and DCT respectively. The experimental results show that the imperceptibility of the watermarked image is acceptable and the method is robust for common signal processing attacks. *The proposed method can be also applied on color images. However, the authors have not considered watermark security problems such as reshaping or visual cryptography before embedding.* Umaamaheshvari and Thanushkodi [24] proposed a frequency domain watermarking method to check the integrity and authenticity of the medical images. In the embedding process, DCT is first applied to the original image to generate a resultant transformed matrix. A hybrid transformed image is obtained next on applying Daubechies 4 wavelet transform on the resultant transformed matrix. Now, the least significant bit (LSB) value of every two bytes of the hybrid transformed image is computed followed by the XOR operation. Furthermore, each pixel value of the binary watermark image is compared with the resultant XOR value to obtain a modified embedded transformed image which is then mapped back to its original position. The extraction process is just reversing the embedding process. The Daubechies 4 wavelet transform technique used by the authors is useful for local analysis but it has higher computational overhead.

Soliman et al. [25] proposed an adaptive watermarking scheme based on swarm intelligence. After the first level decomposition of DWT cover image, DCT is applied only on low frequency components. Now, for each block of DCT coefficient a quantization parameter is determined from HVS by using luminance and texture masks followed by particle swarm optimization (PSO) training. Hajjaji et al. [26] proposed a medical image watermarking method based on DWT and K-L transform. The K-L transform is applied only on sub-bands of the second level DWT of the cover image. A binary signature owned by the hospital center is generated by SHA-1 hash function and rest of the patient record is concatenated with this binary signature. Before embedding the patient record into the cover image, it is coded by the serial turbo code. The method achieved high robustness and good imperceptibility against signal processing attacks. Kannammal and Subha Rani [27] focused on the issue of the security for medical images and proposed an encryption based image watermarking method in frequency and spatial domain. The method uses medical image as watermark which is embedded in the selected DWT sub-band of the cover image. For the watermark embedding, the LSB method is used. After embedding process, the watermarked image is then encrypted. Based on the experimental results, RC4 encryption algorithm was found to perform better than AES and RSA algorithms in terms of encryption/decryption time. The method achieved high robustness and security against signal processing attacks. Al-Haj [28] presented a region based watermarking algorithm for medical images. The method used multiple watermarks (robust and fragile) in spatial (LSB) and frequency domain (DWT and SVD). The robust watermark is embedded in NROI part of the cover image using frequency domain technique to avoid any compromise on its diagnostic value. The fragile watermark is embedded into ROI of the cover image using the spatial domain technique. The method achieved high robustness against JPEG and salt & pepper attacks.

Priya et al. [29] proposed a medical image watermarking method based on spatial and frequency domain embedding. This method uses LSB and DWT, DCT and DFT for watermarking. After transforming the cover image, the image in read in zig-zag manner. Based on the experimental results, DWT provides better performance in term of robustness and imperceptibility than the LSB method. Gao et al. [30] presented a hybrid method for medical image watermarking based on redundancy discrete wavelet transform (RDWT) and SVD. This uses embedding process by applying first level RDWT to the cover image which decomposes the cover image into four sub-bands. Next, SVD is applied on each sub-band. The cover image itself is used as watermark and this method offers high robustness without significant degradation of the image quality against rotation attack. In addition to this, the proposed method has the ability of rotation correction function and high embedding capacity.

Rosiyadi et al. [31] proposed another hybrid watermarking method based on DCT and SVD for the copyright protection. In this embedding process, DCT is applied on the host image using the zigzag space-filling curve (SFC) for the DCT coefficients and subsequently the SVD is applied on the DCT coefficients. Finally, the host image is modified by the left singular vectors and the singular values of the DCT coefficients to embed the watermark image. In this method, genetic algorithm (GA) based technique is used to find the optimization scaling factor of the watermark image. They have experimentally shown that the proposed method is robust against several kinds of attacks. The comparison between the method based on DCT and SVD using GA and the hybrid method based on DCT-SVD has been presented by Rosiyadi et al. in [32]. It is shown that the robustness of the extracted watermark and the visual quality of the watermarked image of the method using GA technique is better than the hybrid method. Horng et al. [33] proposed a blind watermarking method based on DCT, SVD and GA. It is shown that this method is robust and offers high imperceptibility against several known attacks. Horng et al. [34] proposed an adaptive watermarking method based on DCT, SVD and GA. In this embedding process, the host image luminance masking is used and the mask of each sub-band area is transformed into frequency domain. Subsequently, the watermark image is embedded by modifying the singular values of DCT-transformed host image with singular values of mask coefficients of host image and the control parameter of DCT-transformed watermark image using GA. It is shown that this method is robust against several known attacks. A region based robust and secure watermarking method is presented by Sharma et al. [35] for medical applications. The method initially uses DWT and DCT to embeds multiple watermark information in to the cover medical image. Further, the security of the image and text watermark information is enhanced by message-digest (MD5) hash algorithm and Rivest–Shamir–Adleman (RSA) respectively before embedding into the medical cover image. In order to enhance the robustness of the text watermark hamming error correction code is also applied on the encrypted watermark. The experimental results has been shown that the method is robust for important signal processing attacks.

Pandey et al. [36] presents a secure DWT and SVD based multiple watermarking methods for Tele-ophthalmology applications. To enhance the security of the method, secure hash algorithm (SHA-512) is used for generating hash corresponding to iris part of the cover digital eye image. The suggested technique initially divides the digital eye image into Region-of-Interest (ROI) containing iris and Non

Region-of-interest (NROI) part where the text and image watermarks are embedded into the NROI part of the DWT cover image. The performance in terms of Normalized Correlation (NC) and bit error rate (BER) of the developed scheme is evaluated and analyzed against known signal processing attacks and "Checkmark" attacks. The method is found to be robust against all the considered attacks. In [37], the authors present a watermarking method using lifting wavelet transform (LWT) and block based DCT are applied to the cover image followed by the normalizing an image. Further, the DC coefficients from all blocks are gathered and singular value matrix is constructed using SVD. The watermark image is embedded in this singular value matrix after scrambling the image, which increases the security of the proposed scheme.

Potential researchers have proposed image watermarking techniques based on combination of DWT, DCT and SVD [38–44]. Singh and Tayal [38] proposed a hybrid algorithm for image watermarking based on DWT, DCT, and SVD by first decomposing the host and the watermark image into first level DWT. This is followed by transforming both the high frequency band (HH) of the cover image and watermark image using DCT and SVD. The 'S' vector of watermark information is embedded in the 'S' component of the host image. The performance of Haar, Daubechies2, Biorthogonal1.1, and Coiflet1 filters against different signal processing attacks has been evaluated and compared. Khan et al. [39] proposed a hybrid method for image watermarking using DWT, DCT and SVD in a zig-zag order. The proposed method has been extensively tested against known attacks and has been found to give superior performance for robustness and imperceptibility compared to the existing methods based on DCT–SVD or DWT only. Srivastava and Saxena [40] proposed a semi-blind image watermarking method based on DWT, DCT and SVD. In this embedding process, the host and the watermark images are decomposed into first level DWT and then the watermark is transformed by DCT and SVD before embedding it into middle frequency band of the cover image. The method is robust against various attacks. Harish et al. [41] also developed a hybrid method based on DWT, DCT and SVD. This embedding process uses modification of the singular values of the DCT coefficients of the cover image with the singular values of the watermark image. The proposed method is shown to be robust against various attacks. Zear et al. [42] proposed a robust and secure hybrid multiple watermarking technique through discrete wavelet transforms (DWT), discrete cosine transform (DCT) and singular value decomposition (SVD) and neural network using medical images. Two different text watermark information is compressed and encoded by arithmetic and hamming error correction code respectively. The compressed and encoded text watermark is embedding into the cover image. Further, Arnold transform is applied on the image watermark before embedding into the cover. The performance of the algorithm has been extensively evaluated in terms of PSNR, NC and BER.

Singh et al. [43] have presents a secure multiple watermarking method based on DWT, DCT and SVD. For identity authentication purpose, the proposed method uses medical image as the image watermark, and the personal and medical record of the patient as the text watermark. In order to enhance the security of the text watermark, the encryption is applied to the ASCII representation of the text watermark before embedding. The experimental results have shown that the method is robust for various signal processing and "Checkmark' attacks. In order to improve the performance of the method proposed, DWT applied on watermark image instead of DCT as proposed in [44].

2.2.4 Watermarking Using Machine Learning Techniques

Wavelet based image watermarking using machine learning techniques are proposed in [45–70]. Although these proposed methods offer high imperceptibility and robustness but they involve high computational complexity. Peng et al. [45] proposed a blind watermarking method based on multi-wavelet and support vector machine (SVM). In this watermarking process, first level multi-wavelet is performed on each block of image and then the watermark information is embedded into lower frequency sub-band of the cover image using modulation technique. Here, the watermark information consists of two components, a reference information and owner signature of binary logo image. The reference information is used to train SVM during watermark extraction process. Based on experimental results, it is shown that the proposed method achieves high imperceptibility and robustness over other methods [46–48]. However, the computational complexity of this method is higher.

Vafaei et al. [49] proposed a blind watermarking method based on DWT and Artificial Neural Network (ANN). In this watermarking method the third level DWT is applied on the cover image and the binary image watermark is then embedded repetitively into the selected wavelet coefficients. ANN is used to balance between the robustness of the extracted watermark and the quality of the watermarked image. The proposed method offers good imperceptibility and high robustness simultaneously to cropping, filtering and noise addition attacks. However, the time complexity of the method is very high. Sridevi and Fathima [50] proposed a watermarking method based on DWT and using GA and fuzzy inference system to find the embedding strength. In this embedding process, the cover image is decomposed by DWT and the watermark is embedded into the selected sub-band. This method is robust without much degradation of the image quality. The PSNR values of retrieved watermark are very low but the visual quality is good. However, this method is not resistant to the noise attack.

Kang et al. [51] proposed a blind wavelet based watermarking method using Principal Component Analysis (PCA) technique. Their method uses embedding an encrypted watermark image into the main component of the wavelet domain of the cover image. Before embedding the watermark, it is encrypted in order to enhance the security of the watermark information. Wang et al. [52] proposed a blind DWT based watermarking method using neural network where DWT is applied on cover image and weight factors are calculated for the wavelet coefficients and the watermark is then embedded into selected coefficients. The proposed method is tested against JPEG compression attack only (up to 70% quality factor). Tsai et al.

[53] proposed DWT based blind watermarking method using neural network and HVS characteristics wherein noticeable differences profile is employed to embed the watermark. The proposed method has better transparency performance than Joo's et al. [54] and Wang and Pearmain [55] methods.

Ni et al. [56] proposed a watermarking method based on DWT and Hidden Markov Model (HMM) by applying the fourth level DWT on cover image to build vector trees and then the watermark is embedded into designated trees. Before embedding the watermark, it is coded with repeat accumulation error-correcting code. Miyazaki [57] proposed a watermarking detection method based on DWT and Bayesian estimation. Shao et al. [58] proposed a discrete multiwavelet transform (DMWT) based blind watermarking method using SVM in which the cover image is decomposed by DMWT and the watermark is embedded into one of the selected sub-band. Before embedding the watermark, it is transformed by Arnold transformation. This method has better image quality of the watermarked image and robustness of the extracted watermark against number of signal processing attacks than method suggested by Li et al. [59]. Hsieh [60] proposed a watermarking method based on DWT and fuzzy logic based on applying third level DWT on cover image and calculating the entropy of the coefficient. The coefficients with larger entropy are selected for watermark embedding.

Surekha and Sumathi [61] proposed a watermarking method based on DWT and GA. In this embedding process, the cover image is decomposed by DWT and the watermark information is embedded into detail sub-bands of the cover. The method uses GA to optimize the watermark strength factor at every chosen sub-band. Ramanjaneyulu and Rajarajeswari [62] proposed a DWT based watermarking method using GA by applying third level DWT on cover image, selecting suitable sub-bands for watermark embedding and optimization is achieved using GA. This method achieves better imperceptibility and robustness performance than other methods [63–66]. Ramamurthy and Varadarajan [67] proposed two different DWT based image watermarking methods and compared them. The first method is based on neural network and the other method is based on fuzzy logic. They found that the first method is good for filtering attacks whereas the second method is good for cropping, jpeg, rotation and salt and pepper attack.

Dang and Kinsner [68] proposed an image watermarking method based on DWT and neural network wherein the colour image of the cover image is decomposed by DWT using HVS model and then the watermark is embedded into the selected coefficients. Imran and Ghafoor [69] proposed non-blind DWT-SVD based image watermarking method using PCA technique. In this method, the color cover and watermark images are decomposed by DWT and then SVD is applied on the selected sub-band. Subsequently, the singular value of the watermark image is embedded into the singular value of the cover image. Before the embedding process, PCA is used to un-correlate the R (Red), G (Green) and B (Blue) channels of the color cover and watermark image. Mangaiyarkarasi and Arulselvi [70] proposed a medical image watermarking method based on DWT and independent component analysis (ICA). After the second level decomposition of the cover image by DWT, the binary logo watermark is embedded into the selected sub-band of the cover image. The proposed embedding method highly depends on the computation of noise visibility function (NVF). Fast ICA method is used for the watermark extraction process. The proposed method offers high robustness and good image quality against signal processing attacks.

2.2.5 Biometric Watermarking

Use of biometric image as watermark [71, 72] has been proposed to achieve two level security. Selvy et al. [71] proposed watermarking method based on biometrics (Iris), wavelet-based contourlet transform (WBCT) and SVD. In this embedding process, second level decomposition is performed on randomized cover image. The SVD is applied on all the sub-bands of cover and watermark images where the singular value of the host image is modified with the singular value of the watermark image. The iris biometric has high universality, high distinctiveness, high permanence and high performance than the other biometric traits. Also, WBCT contains the directional information of the image which is not provided by DWT. Wioletta [72] proposed a biometric (Iris) based medical image watermarking method using DWT to embed iris watermark into the cover medical image. This method offers high robustness in lower frequency component of DWT cover image against signal processing attacks. The combination of biometric and watermarking methods provides the security solutions to the medical image watermarking. However, noise in sensed data, non-universality, intra class variations and inter class similarity are the some limitations of the biometric based methods.

2.2.6 Joint Compression and Watermarking

In recent time, the transmission and storage of digital documents/information over the unsecured channel is an enormous concern and nearly all of the digital documents are compressed before the document is stored or transmitted to save the bandwidth requirements. As a solution to these, noted researchers are combine the watermarking and compression to addressing the optimal trade-off between major performance parameters including embedding and compression rate, storage space, robustness and embedding alteration against different known signal processing attacks. In order to that Mary et al. [73] proposed an encryption and compression based watermarking method in LSB domain. The cover and watermark image is compressed and encrypted by JPEG 2000 compression technique and modified RC6 block cipher respectively before the embedding process. Further, the encrypted watermark image is embedding into the compressed cover image using LSB to addressing the robustness, capacity and security of the watermarking system. Zargar and Singh [74] proposed a lossy BTC compression based watermarking method in DWT domain. In this paper, BTC compression has been applied on watermark

image before embedding into the cover. The robustness and transparency performance of the proposed method is better than fractal-based compression. Guo and
Liu [75] proposed a joint watermarking and compression technique using BTC. The
method is also addressing the problem of blocking effect and false contour problem
as suffered by BTC. The performance of the proposed method is extensively evaluated by the parameters HVS-PSNR and BER and found to be robust for various
known attacks except JPEG and JPEG2000. Further, the method achieved superior
robustness than other reported techniques [76]. Goudia et al. [77] proposed a robust
joint JPEG 2000 compressing and watermarking technique using DWT and quantization. The experimental results investigated that the method is robust for different
attacks at higher quantization step size with minimum degradation in the visual
quality of the watermarked image.

A lossless compression based watermarking technique is proposed by Badshah
et al. [78] using tele-radiology images. The ROI part of the watermark is considered
along with a key to generate a new watermark. The generated watermark is compressed by LZW technique and the compressed watermark is embedding into the
RONI part of the cover image. The experimental results established that the performance of the different compression method is investigated and found that the LZW
compression technique offer better compression ratio performance than other conventional compression techniques. The method also verifies the tempering in the
watermark after extraction and decompression process. Lin et al. [79] also proposed
a DCT based color image watermarking whereas the watermark information is
embedding into the low frequencies coefficients of the DCT transformed cover
image. The method is robust and imperceptible at different modulus values.

2.2.7 Others Perspectives

Further, some others significant contribution of wavelet based watermarking techniques are proposed by noted researchers in [80–103]. Reddy and Chatterji [80]
suggested a watermarking method to protect the digital watermark where weight
factors for the wavelet coefficients are calculated and the watermark bits are added
to significant coefficients of all DWT sub-bands. In the recovery process, the
extracted watermark bits are combined and normalized. Although this method is
shown to be robust against cropping attack however, the proposed method can detect
noise up to 40% only. Lin and Ching [81] proposed a blind wavelet-based image
hiding method that hides more than one image inside the host image and maintains
the quality of watermarked image. In the watermark embedding process, watermark
image is embedded into low frequency components of the DWT cover image. The
embedded information is scrambled to ensure security and robustness of the watermark simultaneously. The extraction process is same as embedding process but in
reverse order.

Chang et al. [82] have proposed a multipurpose watermarking method based
on integer-DWT (IWT) that achieves both the copyright protection and image

authentication simultaneously. The IWT is easy to implement and has fast multiplication-free implementation. However, the IWT has poor energy compaction than common wavelet transforms. In [83], Yusof and Khalifa have proposed two different watermarking methods. In the first embedding process, first level DWT coefficients of gray-scale watermark is embedded into the second level DWT of the cover image in all sub-bands. However, in the second method, first level DWT coefficients of gray scale watermark are embedded into the second level DWT of the cover image in the selected sub-band. The size of watermark is one fourth the size of cover image. Both methods are robust and offer higher imperceptibility against signal processing attacks.

Yeh et al. [84] have presented a watermarking method that enables ownership protection. After the first level decomposition of the cover image by DWT, watermark information is embedded in the blocks located at the even and odd columns of the high-low (HL) sub-band low-high (LH) sub-band respectively. During embedding the watermark bit, mean value of all four sub-band wavelet coefficients in the block is calculated [85] and modified. The watermark extraction process is just the reverse of the embedding process. The experimental results show that the method is better than the Chang's method [82]. The proposed algorithm can also be applied to color images. Yang and Hu [86] have proposed a watermarking method based on spatial and frequency domain technique. The secret information is embedded in the spatial domain using min-max algorithm to improve the embedding capacity. However, the watermark information is embedded into the selected sub-bands (HL and LH) of the IWT image using coefficient-bias approach. The experimental results indicate that a hidden data can be successfully extracted and a host image can be losslessly restored. Moreover, the resultant perceptual quality generated by the proposed method is good. Kumar et al. [10] proposed a method for telemedicine application based on DWT. The watermark information (doctor's signature) is converted into the binary image and is embedded into the second level decomposition of DWT cover image. Subsequently, two different pseudo-random noise (PN) sequence pairs are generated and the coefficient of chosen sub-band is modified. During the watermark extraction process in this method, same pseudo random matrix is generated which is used during the embedding process of the watermark. The proposed method is robust against the common signal processing attacks. The method is non-blind which requires original image in the recovery process.

Abdallah et al. [87] proposed a blind wavelet-based image watermarking method using quantization of selected wavelet coefficients. After the third level decomposition of the cover image, perceptually significant wavelet coefficients are used to embed the watermark bits. In this method, some wavelet coefficients are selected and assigned as 0 or 1 using quantization process. This process is repeated until all the watermark bits have been recovered. The proposed scheme has better imperceptibility than the Dugad's scheme [88]. Bekkouche and Chouarfia [89] proposed two different image watermarking methods. The first method is the combination of reversible watermarking and code division multiple access (CDMA) in spatial domain, whereas the second method is the combination of reversible watermarking and CDMA in the frequency (DCT and DWT) domain. The experimental results show that the combination of the reversible watermarking and CDMA in DCT domain is more robust against signal processing attacks. The proposed method increases security, authentication, confidentiality and integrity of the image and patient information simultaneously. Although CDMA system has a very high spectral capacity however, the system suffers from self-jamming and near-far problem.

Pal et al. [90] proposed a medical image watermarking method based on DWT. In this method, multiple copies of the same data are embedded into the cover image using bit replacement method. To recover hidden information from the damaged copies, the proposed algorithm finds the closest twin of the embedded information using bit majority algorithm. The experimental results have shown that the proposed algorithm embeds a large payload at a low distortion level. However, the algorithm is inefficient for salt and pepper noise above 40% and JPEG compression above 5%.

Bhatnagar et al. [91] proposed non-blind method based on DWT. In this method, the watermark is embedded in the selected blocks made by zigzag sequence using third level decomposition by DWT of the cover. The blocks are selected based on their variance which further serves as the measure of watermark magnitude that could be imperceptibly embedded in each block. The variance is calculated in a small moving square window process which also computes the mean of the standard deviation values derived for the image. The proposed method is time efficient and robust against signal processing attacks. However, the proposed method is less effective for histogram equalization and wrapping attacks. In [92], a blind watermarking method based on the DWT has been proposed. After the third level decomposition by DWT, the selected sub-bands (LH3) are divided into blocks. In the embedding process, the largest two wavelet coefficients in the block are selected and their significant difference is calculated. After quantizing the maximum wavelet coefficient, the binary watermark bits are embedded into the selected sub-band. During the extraction process, an adaptive threshold value is designed to extract the watermark under different conditions. Experimental results show that the method is robust and the watermarked image quality is good against JPEG compression and low-pass filtering attacks. Lin et al. [93] also proposed a wavelet-tree-based watermarking method using distance vector of binary cluster. In this method, wavelet trees are classified into two clusters using the distance vector to denote binary watermark bits. For embedding, the statistical difference and the distance vector of wavelet tree are compared to select the watermark bits for embedding. The experimental results as reported by authors have shown that the watermarked image quality is very good and the method is robust against known attacks.

Zhang et al. [94] proposed a blind watermarking algorithm based on sparse representation of the compressed sensing (CS) theory and IWT. In this embedding process, IWT is first applied on cover image to obtain the transform coefficients that consist of sparse matrix of image on the row and column followed by a random projection. The histogram shrinkage technology on host image is used to prevent the data overflow. With the help of Arnold transform, scrambled watermark is embedded with the help of IWT and compressed sensing theory. The extraction process is same as embedding but in the reverse order. The proposed method achieved improved robustness and imperceptibility than Lin method [95] and it also enhanced security of the watermark system. However, the algorithm complexity is high.

Wang et al. [96] proposed a semi blind and adaptive watermarking method based on DWT. For the watermark embedding purpose, third level DWT coefficients are categorized into Set Partitioning in Hierarchical Trees (SPIHT). Those trees are further decomposed into a set of bit planes. Now, the binary watermark is embedded into the selected bit planes with adaptive watermark embedding strength. The proposed method is robust and imperceptible against signal processing attacks. Also, the method has good computational efficiency for practical applications. Chen and Zhao [97] developed a robust and blind watermarking technique for 3D images using contourlet transform and depth-image-based rendering (DIBR). The watermark generated through spread spectrum method and each watermark bits is embedding into the selected coefficients of the cover contourlet sub-bands through proper quantization. The PSNR, NC and BER performance of the method is extensively evaluated and found that the low BER performance at different views than other reported methods [98, 99].

Zolotavkin and Juhola [100] proposed a robust watermarking method using QIM. The performance of the method is measured by WNR and document to Watermark Ratio (DWR). The method is found to be robust It provides high robust for additive white Gaussian noise and gain attack. Wang and Allebach [101] proposed a halftone image watermarking in which watermark is embedding into the halftone by using synchronization pattern. The performance of the method is evaluated in terms of PSNR, normalized HVS mean square error and watermark rate and found to be good visual quality and achieved high watermark capacity. An improved spread transform dither modulation based robust and secure watermarking technique was proposed by Cao et al. [102]. The watermark is only embedding into the selected embedding sub-space. The security and robustness performance of the method is extensively evaluated for estimation of projection vector and amplitude scaling attacks respectively. Heidari and Naseri [103] proposed a quantum watermarking method in which quantum signal/information is embedding into the quantum cover image. The method scrambled the watermark information along with the keys are embedding into the cover using LSB technique. The performance is examined in terms of PSNR and authors reported that the method is robust.

Further, Table 2.1 summarizes some inspiring and pioneering robust image watermarking algorithms.

2.3 Potential Challenges and Discussion

The foregoing section presented a detailed review of transform domain specially wavelet based watermarking techniques using ECCs, hybrid techniques, multiple watermarking, biometrics, joint compression and watermarking, machine learning. The analysis of merits and limitations of these techniques with respect to major watermarking benchmark parameters i.e. robustness, imperceptibility, security and

Table 2.1 Summary of inspiring and pioneering robust image watermarking algorithms

Ref. No.	Methodology used	Decomposition level	Cover images/Watermark image	Filter used	Remarks
[1]	DWT, BCH code	Up to third level	MR Image of size 512 × 512/ Maximum size of massage = 381 bits	Haar	– Max PSNR =49.12 dB. – Max BER = 0.0603 against JPEG attacks.
[2]	DWPT, BCH code	Second level	Medical images of size 512 × 512/Massage bits of 2048 bits and watermark logo image of size 128 × 128	Haar	– Radiological image is the more robust against attacks – Obtained PSNR = 39.0999 dB, NC is 1.000 and BER 0.0 without attack.
[9]	Haar Wavelet Quantization Function, BCH, ROI	Fourth level	Medical Images/bit format	Haar	– Addressing health information management Issues – Robust against JPEG attack – Highest PSNR 46.66 – Max BER (%) = 43.6 for MRA image at JPEG (QF = 75). – Normalized hamming distance is determined for different medical images upto fourth level
[11]	Improved robustness using (7,4)-Hamming code, (15,7)-BCH and (15,7)-Reed-Solomon code, DWT	Second Level	Picture of the university/ Maximum size of massage = 360 bits	Haar	– Reed-Solomon code behaves best. – The ECCs considered are not able to deal with error rates greater than 10–20%.
[12]	DWT, SVD, and four different ECCs	Second Level	Medical images of size 512 × 512/Image and text watermark of size 256 × 256 and 20 Characters respectively	Haar	– Hybrid code performed better results in terms of robustness. – Without attacks, max PSNR = 37.22 dB whereas NC = 1 and BER = 0

[13]	IWT, ROI, HVS	First Level	Medical images of size 512 × 512/max massage size of 3400 characters	CDF	– Very good capacity of embedding the watermark – PSNR = 44 dB, WPSNR = 53 dB, BER = 0
[14]	Haar Wavelet Transform	Second Level	Medical image/ECG Signal and patient ID image	Haar	– PSNR = 50 dB, comparison of different wavelet filters
[15]	DWT, spread-spectrum, BCH code	Second	Medical images of size 512 × 512/Health centre logo as image and patient information as text	Haar	– Embedding based on threshold criteria – Health data management – Performance is determined in terms of PSNR, NC and BER
[18]	DCT, DWT	Third Level	Lena image of 256 × 256 / binary image of 32 × 32	LPF, HPF	– PSNR 50.0285 dB and NC is 0.9782 – Robust against attacks.
[21]	DWT, SVD	First	Lena image of 256 × 256 / Cameraman image of 128 × 128	Haar	– PSNR 51.14 dB and max NC 0.9994 – Performance is evaluated in terms of PSNR, NC and efficiency.
[24]	DCT, Daubechies 4 wavelet transform	Fourth Level	Medical image/binary image	Daubechies-4	– PSNR value is 56 to 57 dB and SSIM value is 0.79–0.85.
[25]	Particle swarm optimization, DWT-DCT domain	First Level	Medical images of size 512 × 512/binary bits of size 32 × 32	Haar	– Robust against a wide variety of common attacks
[26]	DWT, KLT, serial Turbocode	Second Level	Radiographic images of size 512 × 512/patient data	Haar	– An initial visibility factor value is determined using Fuzzy Inference System (FIS) – Performance is evaluated in terms of PSNR, WPSNR and NC – Without attacks, the PSNR = 56.8716 dB and WPSNR = 67.7058 dB and NC = 1 when the rate of image compression goes from 10% to 70%.

(continued)

Table 2.1 (continued)

Ref. No.	Methodology used	Decomposition level	Cover images/Watermark image	Filter used	Remarks
[27]	Fusion of watermarking and encryption, LSB methods	First Level	Natural images of size 512 × 512/Medical images	Non-tensor product wavelet filter banks	– Performance of RSA, AES and RC4 is investigated. – RC4 encryption algorithm performs better than AES and RSA algorithms. – Performance is evaluated in terms of PSNR, SSIM, NC, and Correlation Value (CV) – Robust against different attacks
[28]	DWT, SVD, ROI, NROI	First Level	Medical image of 2048 × 2048/patient information and logo	Haar	– Excellent embedding capacity – The algorithm was evaluated with respect to imperceptibility, robustness, capacity, and tamper localization capability. – Extensive use of cryptographic primitives is considered a major limitation of the method. – The embedding time of the watermarks is much higher than the time spent in the extraction process
[31]	DCT, SVD, zigzag SFC, genetic algorithm	Apply DCT on host image	e-government document image of size 256 × 1024/watermark image of size 256 × 256	–	– Avoid the false-positive problem – population size, crossover rate, mutation rate, and generation size, are 30, 0.8, 0.01, and 50, respectively. – Robust against several kinds of attacks

Ref	Techniques	Level	Image/watermark	Transform	Observations
[33]	Joint encryption watermarking, LSB, QIM, RC4	—	Image of 576 × 690/massage along with key	—	– A capacity rate of 1 and 0.5 bits of message per pixel. – Performance is determined in terms of PSNR and Entropy. – PSNR is greater than 49 dB
[35]	DWT, DCT, MD5, RSA, Hamming error correction code, ROI and NROI	Second Level	Medical images of size 512 × 512/Watermark images of size 256 × 256, text watermark of 33 characters	Haar	– Robust against various attacks – Fusion of watermarking and cryptography – Encoding and decoding time is determined for different size of EPR watermark
[36]	DWT, SVD SHA-512, ROI and NROI	Fourth Level	Medical image of size 1024 × 1024/ watermark image of size 512 × 512 and text watermark of size 5145 bits	Haar	– Health data management – Robust against various attacks including checkmark
[42]	DWT, DCT, SVD, BPNN, Arnold transform, arithmetic compression technique, Hamming error correction	Third level	CT-scan image of size 512 × 512/Lump watermark image of size 256 × 256 and text watermark of 190 characters	Haar	– Robust against various kind of attacks – PSNR is evaluated by the subjective method also. – Health data management
[43]	DWT, DCT, SVD, encryption	Second level	Medical image of size 512 × 512/watermark image of size 256 × 256 and text watermark of 50 characters	Haar	– Health data management – Robust against various attacks including checkmark – Performance is calculated in terms of PSNR, NC and BER – Visual quality of the watermarked image is evaluated by the subjective method also

(continued)

Table 2.1 (continued)

Ref. No.	Methodology used	Decomposition level	Cover images/Watermark image	Filter used	Remarks
[44]	DWT, DCT, SVD, encryption	Second Level	Digital image of size 512 × 512/watermark image of size 256 × 256 and text watermark of 185 characters	Haar	– Health data management – Robust against various attacks including checkmark – Performance is calculated in terms of PSNR, NC and BER – Visual quality of the watermarked image is evaluated by the subjective method also
[45]	Multi wavelet, SVM, Modulation technique	First level	Lena, Peppers, Boat/binary logo	–	– PSNR = 42.38, BER = 0–0.3 – Robust against common attacks
[49]	DWT, PCA	Third level	Digital image of size 512 × 512/binary watermark image of size 32 × 32	Haar	– Robust against common attacks
[78]	LZW, ROI	–	ROI size of the cover medical = 100 × 100, secret key length = 64/ uncompressed watermark binary stream = 80,256 values	–	– LZW gives the better compression ratios than other conventional methods
[80]	DWT, HVS characteristics	Fourth Level	Lena of size 512 × 512/gray scale logo of size 64 × 64	Haar	– Robust, detected up to 40% noise
[81]	DWT, Scrambled the Embedded Information	Third Level	Lena and Baboon/digital image of size 512 × 512	Haar	– The method can hide up to three full size images where the PSNR above 32 dB
[89]	Cryptography tools, CDMA in Frequency (DWT, DCT) and Spatial Domain (LSB)	First Level	Medical/gray image	–	– Compared the results on the basis of PSNR, MSE, Mean Absolute Error and SNR

[90]	DWT, Bit Majority method	First level	Medical Images, logo images		– PSNR values are 41.19–42.34 dB and SSIM values are 0.96–0.988 for different images
[91]	DWT, segmentation using ZIG-ZIG sequence	Third level	Gray-scale images of size 256 × 256/8-bit gray scale logo of size 32 × 32	Daubechies	– Max PSNR = 57.74 and embedding and extraction time is 11.07 s – Robust against intentional or un-intentional variety of attacks.
[97]	contourlet transform	First Level	DIBR 3D images	Gaussian filter	– Using Middlebury Stereo Datasets for experimental purpose – Performance is evaluated in terms of PSNR, NC, SSIM, BER, mean opinion score – Robust against Geometric Attacks
[113]	DDM based on CSF filter, LSB, DWT	Second Level	Fundus image/Text data	CSF filter	– Performance comparable with the standard PSNR

IWT integer wavelet Transform, *DWT* discrete wavelet transform, *PSNR* peak signal-to-noise-ratio, *DCT* discrete cosine transform, *ROI* Region-of-interest, *CSF* contrast sensitive function, *SST* spread-spectrum technique, *HM* histogram modification, *LPF* low pass filter, *HPF* high pass filter, *WPSNR* weighted peak signal to noise ratio, *CDF* Cohen-Daubechies Feauveau, *BER* bit error rate, *NC* normalized cross-correlation, *DWPT* discrete wavelet packet transform, *PCA* principal component analysis, *CDMA* code division multiple access, *GA* genetic algorithm, *SFC* space-filling curve, *QIM* quantization index modulation, *DIBR* depth-image-based rendering, *LZW* Lempel–Ziv–Welch, *LSB* least substitution bit, *KLT* Karhunen-Loeve transform capacity revealed that it is difficult to achieve satisfactory performance with respect to imperceptibility, robustness, embedding capacity and security simultaneously. Therefore, it is clear that there are different methods for improving one or a subset of these parameters but they compromise with other remaining parameters. Thus, there is need to develop effective watermarking methods that can offer optimum trade-off between these parameters for telemedicine application. Further, medical image watermarking for telemedicine necessarily requires watermark security against different attacks. Besides this, computational cost of watermarking is also an important parameter to determine the suitability of the watermarking technique. Some important investigations by the authors in the area of medical image watermarking are:

1. *Security of the watermarks*: Most of the medical watermarking methods fall short of this requirement [104, 105]. Some digital watermarking will not need any security because there is hardly any stimulus to disrupt the watermark but others require security against attacks of different kinds. Various researches have been done in recent years to create medical watermark systems which are secure against active attack [27, 106–108]. However, spread spectrum [1, 10, 22, 102] and biometric watermarking [48], or multimodal biometric watermarking security mechanisms [109, 110] are be considered to enhance the security of the watermark. In addition, for the security issues, encrypting EPR data before watermarking has become unavoidable, but the delay encountered during embedding and extraction of the watermark is also an important factor in telemedicine applications [12, 43]. Therefore, watermark constitution by using encryption methods should be simple to save execution time. Recently, the speed has become an important factor if the situation demands in some important applications such as tele-diagnosis and telemedicine.

2. *Selection of ROI and NROI part for embedding watermark*: Any image comprises of two sections called ROI and NROI [35]. ROI is an area that has sensitive data, so it cannot be allowed to be modified because most of the information is present in this area [105]. NROI is an area of image that does not have an important data i.e. background of image. The proper selection of NROI for watermarking is crucial for example in medical images where the area under concern has to be the least required portion conveying any information. It will give better protection if the data is embedded outside of ROI [111, 112].

3. *Selection of DWT sub-bands for embedding watermark*: The selection of sub-bands for embedding watermark is a challenge as it affects robustness against various types of attacks. It has been proved that embedding the watermark in diagonal sub-band coefficients is more robust as compared to horizontal and vertical coefficients [105, 113]. There is no need to have knowledge on the coefficients selected for data embedding when pseudo bits are also embedded [81, 82]. Also, watermark embedding into color image provides greater space against the

watermark embedding into gray scale image. This space will hide more water-mark information [114].

4. *Embedding more than one watermark into cover media*: Huge amount of band-width is required for the transmission of the image data for telemedicine pur-poses. The addition requirement of bandwidth for the transmission of the metadata can be avoided if the data is hidden in the image itself [9, 15]. Since the EPR and the image embedded into one, bandwidth for the transmission can be reduced in telemedicine applications. However, this will increase the computa-tional cost of the watermarking method.

5. *Improve the robustness of extracted watermark*: Various noted researchers are using error correcting codes [1, 2, 9, 11, 12], hybrid techniques [16–44], machine learning techniques [45–70], and some other novel perspectives [80–103] meth-ods to improved the robustness of the extracted watermark(s). However, these methods are compromising with other performance parameters of the water-marking systems. Further, use of ECC for digital watermarking is still an open problem [105].

6. *Simultaneous compression and watermarking*: The medical/digital images require a huge amount of memory in original form and thus there is a need for compression in data hiding [115]. It has been observed that the JPEG/JPEG200 compression which is applied on majority of the digital information/data to reduce the bandwidth requirements during transmission is one of the most com-mon and unavoidable attacks to watermarking systems [75, 77, 116]. In order to achieve the goals of green computing and low delay, some of the researchers have been studying combined watermarking and compression using quantization in theoretical point of view [117, 118]. Simultaneous compression and water-marking is one of the robust techniques to combat piracy attacks [75]. Medical applications may consider using combined watermarking and compression algo-rithm to improve the performance.

2.4   Summary

This chapter has presented state-of-the-art in the field of medical image watermark-ing techniques. Novel and improved medical image watermarking techniques are invented regularly which are addressing the health data management issues and preventing the medical related identity theft. Based on the extensive review, we have noticed that numerous watermarking techniques are designed for specific applica-tions, while the others are not well established yet but have a great potential. This necessitates development of robust and secure watermarking methods to protect integrity and confidentiality of patient's crucial medical data against unauthorized access and tampering.

References

1. A.K. Singh, B. Kumar, M. Dave, A. Mohan, Robust and imperceptible spread-spectrum watermarking for telemedicine applications. Proc. Natl. Acad. Sci., India Sect. A: Phys. Sci. **85**(2), 295–301 (2015). doi:10.1007/s40010-014-0197-6
2. S.A.K. Mostafa, N. El-sheimy, A.S. Tolba, F.M. Abdelkader, H.M. Elhindy, Wavelet packets-based blind watermarking for medical image management. Open Biomed. Eng. J. **4**, 93–98 (2010)
3. A. Al-Haj, Providing integrity, authenticity, and confidentiality for header and pixel data of DICOM images. J. Digit. Imaging **28**(2), 179–187 (2015)
4. H.-M. Chao, C.-M. Hsu, S. Miaou, A data-hiding technique with authentication, integration, and confidentiality for electronic patient records. IEEE Trans. Inf. Technol. Biomed. **6**(1), 46–53 (2002)
5. G. Coatrieux, H. Maitre, B. Sankur, Y. Rolland, R. Collorec, Relevance of watermarking in medical imaging, in Proceedings of the IEEE EMBS Conference on Information Technology Applications in Biomedicine, Arlington, USA, pp. 250–255, 2000
6. G. Coatrieux, L. Lecornu, Ch. Roux, B. Sankur, A review of image watermarking applications in healthcare, in Proceedings of IEEE-EMBC Conference, New York, USA, pp. 4691–4694, 2006
7. U.R. Acharya, D. Anand, P.S. Bhat, U.C. Niranjan, Compact storage of medical images with patient information. IEEE Trans. Inf. Technol. Biomed. **5**(4), 320–323 (2001)
8. A. Giakoumaki, S. Pavlopoulos, D. Koutsouris, A medical image watermarking scheme based on wavelet transform, in Proceedings of 25th Annual International Conference of IEEE-EMBS, San Francisco, pp. 1541–1544, 2004
9. A. Giakoumaki, S. Pavlopoulos, D. Koutsouris, Secure and efficient health data management through multiple watermarking on medical images. Med. Biol. Eng. Comput. **44**, 619–631 (2006)
10. B. Kumar, H.V. Singh, S.P. Singh, A. Mohan, Secure spread spectrum watermarking for telemedicine applications. J. Inf. Secur. **2**, 91–98 (2011)
11. N. Terzija, M. Repges, K. Luck, W. Geisselhardt, Digital image watermarking using discrete wavelet transform: performance comparison of error correction codes, in Proceedings of International Association of Science and Technology for Development, 2002
12. A.K. Singh, B. Kumar, M. Dave, A. Mohan, Robust and imperceptible dual watermarking for telemedicine applications. Wirel. Pers. Commun. **80**(4), 1415–1433 (2014)
13. K.A. Navas, S.A. Thampy, M. Sasikumar, ERP hiding in medical images for telemedicine, in Proceedings of World Academy of Science and Technology, vol. 28, pp. 266–269, 2008
14. A. Kannammal, K. Pavithra, S. SubhaRani, Double watermarking of DICOM medical images using wavelet decomposition technique. Eur. J. Sci. Res. **70**(1), 55–46 (2012)
15. A.K. Singh, B. Kumar, M. Dave, A. Mohan, Multiple watermarking on medical images using selective DWT coefficients. J. Med. Imaging Health Inf. **5**(3), 607–614 (2015)
16. D.-Ch. Lou, Ch.-H. Sung, Robust image watermarking based on hybrid transformation, in Proceedings of IEEE International Carnahan Conference on Security Technology, Taiwan, pp. 394–399, 2003
17. Md. Ouhsain, E.E. Abdallah, A.B. Hamza, An image watermarking scheme based on wavelet and multiple-parameter fractional Fourier transform, in Proceedings of IEEE International Conference on Signal Processing and Communications, Dubai, United Arab Emirates, pp. 1375–1378, 2007
18. M. Jiansheng, L. Sukang, T. Xiaomei, A digital watermarking algorithm based on DCT and DWT, in Proceedings of International Symposium on Web Information Systems and Applications, Nanchang, P.R. China, pp. 104–107, 2009
19. A.S. Hadi, B.M. Mushgil, H.M. Fadhil, Watermarking based Fresnel transform, wavelet transform, and chaotic sequence. J. Appl. Sci. Res. **5**(10), 1463–1468 (2009)

20. C. Cao, R. Wang, M. Huang, R. Chen, A new watermarking method based on DWT and Fresnel diffraction transforms, in Proceedings of IEEE International Conference on Information Theory and Information Security, Beijing, pp. 433–430, 2010
21. C.-C. Lai, C.-C. Tsai, Digital image watermarking using discrete wavelet transform and singular value decomposition. IEEE Trans. Instrum. Meas. 59(11), 3060–3063 (2010)
22. A.A. Nakhaie, S.B. Shokouhi, No reference medical image quality measurement based on spread spectrum and discrete wavelet transform using ROI processing, in Proceedings of 24th Canadian Conference on Electrical and Computer Engineering, pp. 121–125, 2011
23. V.K. Ahire, V. Kshirsagar, Robust watermarking scheme based on discrete wavelet transform (DWT) and discrete cosine transform (DCT) for copyright protection of digital images. IJCSNS 11(8), 208–213 (2011)
24. A. Umaamaheshvari, K. Thanushkodi, High performance and effective watermarking scheme for medical images. Eur. J. Sci. Res. 67(2), 283–293 (2012)
25. M. Soliman, A.E. Hassanien, N.I. Ghali, H.M. Onsi, An adaptive watermarking approach for medical imaging using swarm intelligent. Int. J. Smart Home 6(1), 37–50 (2012)
26. M.A. Hajjaji, E.-B. Bourennane, A.B. Abdelali, A. Mtibaa, Combining Haar wavelet and Karhunen Loeve transforms for medical images watermarking. Biomed. Res. Int. 2014, 1–15 (2014)
27. A. Kannammal, S. Subha Rani, Two level security for medical images using watermarking/ encryption algorithms. Int. J. Imaging Syst. Technol. 24(1), 111–120 (2014)
28. A. Al-Haj, A. Amer, Secured telemedicine using region-based watermarking with tamper localization. J. Digit. Imaging 27(6), 737–750 (2014)
29. S. Priya, B. Santhi, P. Swaminathan, Study on medical image watermarking techniques. J. Appl. Sci. 14(14), 1638–1642 (2014)
30. L. Gao, T. Gao, G. Sheng, S. Zhang, Robust medical image watermarking scheme with rotation correction, in Intelligent Data Analysis and Its Applications, Vol. 2, Advances in Intelligent Systems and Computing, ed. by J.-S. Pan et al. (Eds), vol. 298, (Springer, New York, 2014), pp. 283–292
31. D. Rosiyadi, S.-J. Horng, P. Fan, X. Wang, Copyright protection for e-government document images. IEEE Multimedia 19(3), 62–73 (2012)
32. D. Rosiyadi, S.-J. Horng, N. Suryana, N. Masthurah, A comparison between the hybrid using genetic algorithm and the pure hybrid watermarking scheme. Int. J. Comput. Theory Eng. 4(3), 329–331 (2012)
33. S.-J. Horng, D. Rosiyadi, T. Li, T. Takao, M. Guo, M.K. Khan, A blind image copyright protection scheme for e-government. J. Vis. Commun. Image Represent. 24(7), 1099–1105 (2013)
34. S.-J. Horng, D. Rosiyadi, P. Fan, X. Wang, M.K. Khan, An adaptive watermarking scheme for e-government document images. Multimedia Tools Appl. 72(3), 3085–3103 (2014)
35. A. Sharma, A.K. Singh, S.P. Ghrera, Robust and secure multiple watermarking technique for medical images. Wirel. Pers. Commun. 92(4), 1611–1624 (2017)
36. R. Pandey, A.K. Singh, B. Kumar, A. Mohan, Iris based secure NROI multiple eye image watermarking for teleophthalmology. Multimedia Tools Appl. 75, 14381 (2016). doi:10.1007/ s11042-016-3536-6
37. Y. Niu, X. Cui, Q. Li, J. Ding, A SVD-based color image watermark algorithm in DWT domain, in Advanced Graphic Communications, Packaging Technology and Materials, Lecture Notes in Electrical Engineering, vol. 369, (Springer, New York, 2015), pp. 303–309
38. A. Singh, A. Tayal, Choice of wavelet from wavelet families for DWT–DCT–SVD image watermarking. Int. J. Comput. Appl. 48(17), 9–14 (2012)
39. M.I. Khan, M.M. Rahman, M.I.H. Sarker, Digital watermarking for image authentication based on combined DCT, DWT, and SVD transformation. Int. J. Comput. Sci. 10(5), 223–230 (2013)
40. A. Srivastava, P. Saxena, DWT-DCT-SVD based semi blind image watermarking using middle frequency band. IOSR J. Comput. Eng. 12(2), 63–66 (2013)

41. N.J. Harish, B.B.S. Kumar, A. Kusagur, Hybrid robust watermarking techniques based on DWT, DCT, and SVD. Int.J. Adv. Electr. Electron. Eng. **2**(5), 137–143 (2013)
42. A. Zear, A.K. Singh, P. Kumar, A proposed secure multiple watermarking technique based on DWT, DCT and SVD for application in medicine. Multimedia Tools Appl. (2016). doi:10.1007/s11042-016-3862-8
43. A.K. Singh, M. Dave, A. Mohan, Hybrid technique for robust and imperceptible multiple watermarking using medical images. Multimedia Tools Appl. **75**(14), 8381–8401 (2016)
44. A.K. Singh, Improved hybrid technique for robust and imperceptible multiple watermarking using medical images. Multimedia Tools Appl. **76**, 8881–8900 (2016). doi:10.1007/s11042-016-3514-z
45. H. Peng, J. Wang, W. Wang, Image watermarking method in multiwavelet domain based on support vector machines. J. Syst. Softw. **83**, 1470–1477 (2010)
46. G.D. Fu, H. Peng, Sub sampling-based wavelet watermarking algorithm using support vector regression, in Proceedings of EUROCON, Warsaw, pp. 9–12, 2007
47. J. Zhang, N.-C. Wang, F. Xiong, Hiding a logo watermark into the multiwavelet domain using neural networks, in Proceedings of 14th IEEE International Conference on Tools with Artificial Intelligence, pp. 477–482, 2002
48. H.-H. Tsai, D.-W. Sun, Color image watermark extraction based on support vector machines. Inf. Sci. **177**(2), 550–569 (2007)
49. M. Vafaei, H. Mahdavi-Nasab and H. Pourghassem (2013) A new robust blind watermarking method based on neural networks in wavelet transform domain, World Appl. Sci. J., Vo. 22, No. 11, pp. 1572–1580.
50. T. Sridevi, S.S. Fathima, Watermarking algorithm using genetic algorithm and HVS. Int. J. Comput. Appl. **74**(13), 26–30 (2013)
51. X. Kang, W. Zeng, J. Huang, X. Zhuang, Y.-Q. Shi, Digital watermarking based on multi-band wavelet and principal component analysis. Proc. SPIE **5960**, 1–7 (2005)
52. Z. Wang, N. Wang, B. Shi, A novel blind watermarking scheme based on neural network in wavelet domain, in Proceedings of the 6th Word Congress on Intelligent Control and Automation, Dallan, Chaina, pp. 3024–3027, 2006
53. H.-H. Tsai, C.-C. Liu, K.-C. Wang, Blind wavelet based image watermarking based on HVS and neural networks, in Proceeding of the Joint Conference on Information Sciences, Kaohsiung, Taiwan, 2006
54. S. Joo, Y. Suh, J. Shin, H. Kikuchi, A new robust watermark embedding into wavelet DC components. ETRI J. **24**(5), 401–404 (2002)
55. Y. Wang, A. Pearmain, Blind image data hiding based on self reference. Pattern Recogn. Lett. **25**(15), 1681–1689 (2004)
56. J. Ni, C. Wang, J. Huang, R. Zhang, Performance enhancement for DWT-HMM image watermarking with content-adaptive approach, in Proceeding of International Conference on Image Processing, pp. 1377–1380, 2006
57. A. Miyazaki, Improvement of watermark detection process based on bayesian estimation, in 18th European Conference on Circuit Theory and Design, pp. 408–411, 2007
58. Y. Shao, W. Chen, C. Liu, Multiwavelet based digital watermarking with support vector machine technique, in Control and Decision Conference, pp. 4557–4561, 2008
59. C.-h. Li, Z.-d. Lu, K. Zhou, An image watermarking technique based on support vector regression, in Proceeding of International Symposium Communications and Information Technology, vol. 1, pp. 183–186, 2005
60. M.-S. Hsieh, Perceptual copyright protection using multiresolution wavelet-based watermarking and fuzzy logic. Int. J. Artif. Intell. Appl. **1**(3), 45–57 (2010)
61. P. Surekha, S. Sumathi, Implementation of genetic algorithm for a dwt based image watermarking scheme. ICTACT J. Soft Comput. **2**(1), 244–252 (2011)
62. K. Ramanjaneyulu, K. Rajarajeswari, Wavelet-based oblivious image watermarking scheme sing genetic algorithm. IET Image Process. **6**(4), 364–373 (2012)

63. W.-H. Lin, Y.-R. Wang, S.-J. Horng, A wavelet-tree based watermarking method using distance vector of binary cluster. Expert Syst. Appl. **36**(6), 9869–9878 (2009)
64. S.H. Wang, Y.P. Lin, Wavelet tree quantization for copyright protection watermarking. IEEE Trans. Image Process. **13**(2), 154–165 (2004)
65. E. Li, H. Liang, X. Niu, An integer wavelet based multiple logo-watermarking scheme, in Proceedings of the IEEE WCICA, pp. 10256–10260, 2006
66. B.K. Lien, W.H. Lin, A watermarking method based on maximum distance wavelet tree quantization, in Proceeding of 19th Conference on Computer Vision, Graphics and Image Processing, pp. 269–276, 2006
67. N. Ramamurthy, S. Varadarajank, Robust digital image watermarking scheme with neural network and fuzzy logic approach. Int. J. Emerg. Technol. Adv. Eng. **2**(9), 555–562 (2012)
68. H.V. Dang, W. Kinsner, An intelligent digital colour image watermarking approach based on wavelets and general regression neural networks, in Proceeding of 11th IEEE International Conference on Cognitive Informatics and Cognitive Computing, Kyoto, pp. 115–123, 2012
69. Md. Imran, A. Ghafoor, A PCA-DWT-SVD based color image watermarking, in Proceeding of International Conference on Systems, Man, and Cybernetics, COEX, Seoul, Korea, pp. 1147–1152, 2012
70. P. Mangaiyarkarasi, S. Arulselvi, Medical image watermarking based on DWT and ICA for copyright protection, in *Recent Advancements in System Modelling Applications*, Lecture Notes in Electrical Engineering, ed. by R. Malathi, J. Krishnan (Eds), vol. 188, (Springer, New York, 2013), pp. 21–33
71. P.T. Selvy, V. Palanisamy, E. Soundar, A novel biometrics triggered watermarking of images based on wavelet based Contourlet transform. Int. J. Comput. Appl. Inf. Technol. **2**(2), 19–24 (2013)
72. W. Wioletta, Biometric watermarking for medical images—example of Iris code. Tech. Trans. **1-M**(5), 409–416 (2013)
73. S.J. Jereesha Mary, C. Seldev Christopher, S. Sebastin Antony Joe, Novel scheme for compressed image authentication using LSB watermarking and EMRC6 encryption. Circuits Syst. **7**, 1722–1733 (2016)
74. A. Javeed Zargar, A.K. Singh, Robust and imperceptible image watermarking in DWT-BTC domain. Int. J. Electron. Secur. Digit. Forensics **8**(1), 53–62 (2016)
75. J.-M. Guo, Y.-F. Liu, Joint compression/watermarking scheme using majority parity guidance and half toning-based block truncation coding. IEEE Trans. Image Process. **19**(8), 2056–2069 (2010)
76. M.H. Lin, C.C. Chang, A novel information hiding scheme based on BTC. Proc. Int. Conf. Comput. Inf. Technol. **14–16**, 66–71 (2004)
77. D. Goudia, M. Chaumont, W. Puech, N.H. Said, A joint JPEG2000 compression and watermarking system using a TCQ-based quantization scheme. Vis. Inf. Process. Commun. **II**(VIPC 2011), 78820C–78820C (2011)
78. G. Badshah, S.-C. Liew, J. Md Zain, M. Ali, Watermark compression in medical image watermarking using Lempel-Ziv-Welch (LZW) lossless compression technique. J. Digit. Imaging **29**(2), 216–225 (2016)
79. S.D. Lin, S.-C. Shie, J.Y. Guo, Improving the robustness of DCT-based image watermarking against JPEG compression. Comput. Stand. Interfaces **32**(1–2), 54–60 (2010)
80. A. Reddy, B.N. Chatterji, A new wavelet based logo-watermarking scheme. Pattern Recogn. Lett. **26**(7), 1019–1027 (2005)
81. C.-Y. Lin, C. Yu-Tai, A robust image hiding method using wavelet technique. J. Inf. Sci. Eng. **22**(1), 163–174 (2006)
82. C.C. Chang, W.L. Tai, C.C. Lin, A multipurpose wavelet based image watermarking, in Proceedings of international conference on innovative computing, information and control, Beijing, pp. 70–73, 2006
83. Y. Yusof, O.O. Khalifa, Imperceptibility and robustness analysis of DWT-based digital image watermarking, in International Conference on Computer and Communication Engineering, Kuala Lumpur, Malaysia, pp. 1325–1330, 2008

84. J.P. Yeh, C.-W. Lu, H.-J. Lin, H.-H. Wu, Watermarking technique based on DWT associated with embedding rule. Int. J. Circuits, Syst. Signal Process. **4**(2), 72–82 (2010)
85. C.-Y. Lin, Y.-T. Ching, A robust image hiding method using wavelet technique. J. Inf. Sci. Eng. **22**, 163–174 (2006)
86. C.-Y. Yang, W.-C. Hu, Reversible data hiding in the spatial and frequency domains. Int. J. Image Process. **3**(6), 373–382 (2010)
87. H.A. Abdallah, M.M. Hadhoud, A.A. Shaalan, F.E.A. El-samie, Blind wavelet-based image watermarking. Int. J. Signal Process. Image Process. Pattern Recogn. **4**(1), 15–28 (2011)
88. R. Dugad, K. Ratakonda, N. Ahuja, A new wavelet-based scheme for watermarking images, in Proceeding of the IEEE International Conference on Image Processing, Chicago, IL, USA, pp. 419–423, 1998
89. S. Bekkouche, A. Chouarfia, A new watermarking approach–combined RW/CDMA in spatial and frequency domain. Int. J. Comput. Sci. Telecommun. **2**(4), 1–8 (2011)
90. K. Pal, G. Ghosh, M. Bhattacharya, Biomedical image watermarking in wavelet domain for data integrity using bit majority algorithm and multiple copies of hidden information. Am. J. Biomed. Eng. **2**(2), 29–37 (2012)
91. G. Bhatnagar, Q.M.J. Wu, B. Raman, Robust gray-scale logo watermarking in wavelet domain. Comput. Electr. Eng. **38**(5), 1164–1176 (2012)
92. W.-H. Lin, S.-J. Horng, T.-W. Kao, P. Fan, C.-L. Lee, P. Yi, An efficient watermarking method based on significant difference of wavelet coefficient quantization. IEEE Trans. Multimedia **10**(5), 746–757 (2008)
93. W.-H. Lin, Y.-R. Wang, S.-J. Horng, A wavelet-tree-based watermarking method using distance vector of binary cluster. Expert Syst. Appl. **36**(6), 9869–9878 (2009)
94. Q. Zhang, Y. Sun, Y. Yan, H. Liu, Q. Shang, Research on algorithm of image reversible watermarking based on compressed sensing. J. Inf. Comput. Sci. **10**(3), 701–709 (2013)
95. W.J. Lin, Reconstruction algorithms for compressive sensing and their applications to digital watermarking, Beijing Jiaotong University, Beijing, 2011
96. S. Wang, D. Zheng, J. Zhao, Adaptive watermarking and tree structure based image quality estimation. IEEE Trans. Multimedia **16**(2), 311–325 (2014)
97. Lei Chen and Jiying Zhao, Robust Contourlet-based watermarking for depth-image-based rendering 3D images, 2016 IEEE International Symposium on Broadband Multimedia Systems and Broadcasting (BMSB), Nara, Japan, pp. 1-4.
98. Y.H. Lin, J.L. Wu, A digital blind watermarking for depth-image based rendering 3D images. IEEE Trans. Broadcast. **57**, 602–611 (2011)
99. H.D. Kim, J.W. Lee, T.W. Oh, H.K. Lee, Robust DT-CWT watermarking for DIBR 3D images. IEEE Trans. Broadcast. **58**, 533–543 (2012)
100. Y. Zolotavkin, M. Juhola, A new scalar quantization method for digital image watermarking. J. Electr. Comput. Eng. **2016**, 1–16 (2016)
101. F. Wang, J.P. Allebach, Printed image watermarking using direct binary search Halftoning, in IEEE International Conference on Image Processing, pp. 2727–2731, 2016
102. J. Cao, H. Li, W. Luo, J. Huang, An improved spread transform dither modulation for robust and secure watermarking, in IEEE International Conference on Image Processing, pp. 2718–2722, 2016
103. S. Heidari, M. Naseri, A Novel LSB based quantum watermarking. Int. J. Theor. Phys. **55**(10), 4205–4218 (2016)
104. A.K. Singh, B. Kumar, M. Dave, S.P. Ghrera, A. Mohan, Digital image watermarking: techniques and emerging applications, in *Handbook of Research on Modern Cryptographic Solutions for Computer and Cyber Security*, (IGI Global, USA, 2016), pp. 246–272. doi:10.4018/978-1-5225-0105-3.ch011
105. A.K. Singh, M. Dave, A. Mohan, Wavelet based image watermarking: futuristic concepts in information security. Proc. Natl. Acad. Sci., India Sect. A: Phys. Sci. **84**(3), 345–359 (2014)

106. F. Cayre, C. Fontaine, T. Furon, Watermarking security: theory and practice. IEEE Trans. Signal Process. **53**(10), 3976–3987 (2005)
107. L.P. Freire, P. Comesana, J.R.T. Pastoriza, F.P. Gonzalez, Watermarking security: a survey, in *Transactions on Data Hiding Multimedia Security*, Lecture Notes in Computer Sciences, vol. 4300, (Springer, New York, 2006), pp. 41–72
108. Y.-S. Seo, M.-S. Kim, H.J. Park, H.-Y. Jung, H.-Y. Chung, Y. Hug, J.-D. Lee, A secure watermarking for JPEG2000. Int. Conf. Image Process. **2**, 530–533 (2001)
109. M. Vatsa, R. Singh, A. Noore, Feature based RDWT watermarking for multimodal biometric system. Image Vis. Comput. **27**(3), 293–304 (2009)
110. A.K. Jain, U. Uludag, Hiding Biometric Data. IEEE Trans. Pattern Anal. Mach. Intell. **25**(11), 1494–1498 (2003)
111. J. Zain, M. Clarke, Security in telemedicine: issue in watermarking medical images, in International Conference: Science Of Electronic, Technologies of Information and Telecommunications, 2005
112. N.A. Memon, S.A.M. Gilani, NROI watermarking of medical images for content authentication, in Proceedings of 12th IEEE International Multitopic Conference, Karachi, Pakistan, pp. 106–110, 2008
113. S. Dandapat, J. Xu, O. Chutatape, S.M. Krishnan, Wavelet transform domain data embedding in a medical image, in Proceedings 26th Annual International Conference of IEEE-EMBS, San Francisco, CA, USA, pp. 1541–1544, 2004
114. R. Ridzon, D. Levicky, Content protection in gray scale and color images based on robust digital watermarking. Telecommun. Syst. **52**(3), 1617–1631 (2011)
115. S.P. Nanavati, P.K. Panigrahi, Wavelets: applications to image compression-I. Resonance **10**(2), 52–61 (2005)
116. Y. Zhou, Joint robust watermarking and image compression, in IEEE International Workshop on Information Forensics and Security, WA, USA, pp. 1–6, 2010
117. Y. Zhou, E.-H. Yang, Joint robust watermarking and compression using variable-rate scalar quantization, in Proceedings of The 11th Canadian Workshop on Information Theory, Ottawa, Canada, 2009
118. L. Guillemot, J. Moureaux, Indexing lattice vectors in a joint watermarking and compression scheme, in IEEE International Conference on Acoustics, Speech, Signal Processing, Toulouse, France, 2006

Chapter 3
Analytical Study and Performance Evaluation of Medical Image Watermarking Techniques

Amit Kumar Singh, Basant Kumar, Ghanshyam Singh, and Anand Mohan

3.1 Introduction

As depicted in Fig. 1.2 of Chap. 1, according to working/image domain, the watermark could be applied in spatial and transform domain. The spatial domain techniques such as LSB substitutions, correlation-based, spread-spectrum and Patchwork are straight forward and computationally simple. In this technique the watermark data is embedded directly by manipulating the pixel values, bit stream or code values of the host signal (cover media). However, the spatial domain techniques offer less robustness against the signal processing attacks. In the transform domain techniques, the data is embedded by modulating the coefficients of a transform discrete wavelet transform (DWT), discrete cosine transform (DCT), singular value decomposition (SVD) and discrete Fourier transform (DFT). However, the transform domain watermarking techniques are computationally complex but they provide better robustness of watermarked data.

A.K. Singh (✉)
Department of Computer Science & Engineering, Jaypee University of Information
Technology, Waknaghat, Solan, India
e-mail: amit_245singh@yahoo.com

B. Kumar
Department of Electronics and Communication Engineering, Motilal Nehru National
Institute of Technology, Allahabad, India
e-mail: singhbasant@yahoo.com

G. Singh
Department of Electronics and Communication Engineering, Jaypee University
of Information Technology, Waknaghat, Solan, India
e-mail: drghanshyam.singh@yahoo.com

A. Mohan
Department of Electronics Engineering, Indian Institute of Technology (BHU), Varanasi, India
e-mail: profanandmohan@gmail.com

© Springer International Publishing AG 2017
A.K. Singh et al. (eds.), *Medical Image Watermarking*, Multimedia Systems
and Applications, DOI 10.1007/978-3-319-57699-2_3

3.2 Spatial Domain Techniques

In the spatial domain techniques [1–5], the data is embedded directly by modifying the pixel values of the cover media. The most straightforward way to append a watermark to an image in the spatial domain technique is to add a pseudorandom noise pattern to the luminance values of its pixels [6]. The spatial domain techniques are unable to transfer the protected images to transform domain, and hence these techniques can reduce the computation time of watermark embedding and extraction process. However, the spatial domain techniques are less robust against signal processing attacks. The important spatial domain techniques are presented below.

3.2.1 Least Substitution Bit (LSB)

In all the available watermarking techniques, the least substitution bit (LSB) is the most simple and straight-forward technique [2]. In this technique, the hiding information in a sequence of binary numbers is replacing the LSB of every element with one bit of the secret message. In floating point arithmetic, the least significant bit of the mantissa can be used instead. Since, in general, the size of hidden message is much less than the number of bits available to hide the information rest of the LSB can be left unchanged. However, LSB substitution despite its simplicity has a number of drawbacks. Although it may survive transformations such as cropping, any addition of noise or lossy compression is likely to defeat the watermark. Furthermore, once the algorithm is discovered, the embedded watermark could be easily modified by an intermediate party.

3.2.2 Correlation-Based Technique

This watermarking technique exploits the correlation properties of additive pseudo-random noise patterns as applied to an image [6, 7]. A pseudo-random noise (PN) pattern $W(x,y)$ is added to the cover image $I(x,y)$, according to the Equation shown below.

$$I_w(x,y) = I(x,y) + k \times W(x,y) \tag{3.1}$$

where 'k' denotes a gain factor, and 'I_w' the resulting watermarked image. The robustness of the watermark increases with increase of 'k' at the expense of quality of the watermarked image. To retrieve the watermark, the same pseudo-random noise generator algorithm is seeded with the same key, and the correlation between the noise pattern and possibly watermarked image is evaluated. If the correlation exceeds a certain threshold T, the watermark is detected, and a single bit is set. This technique can easily be extended to a multiple-bit watermark by dividing the image into blocks, and performing the aforementioned procedure independently on each block.

3.2.3 Spread-Spectrum Technique

It is important to know that the watermark should not be placed in insignificant regions of the cover image or its spectrum, since many common signal and geometric processes affect these components. The problem then becomes how to insert a watermark into the most perceptually significant regions of the spectrum while preserving fidelity. Clearly, any spectral coefficient may be altered, provided such modification is small. However, very small changes are very susceptible to noise. This problem can be addressed by applying spread-spectrum watermarking, which can be easily understood with spread-spectrum communication analogy in which the frequency domain of image is viewed as a communication channel, and correspondingly, the watermark is viewed as a signal that is transmitted through it [8]. The immersed signal must be immune to the attacks and unintentional signal distortions (treated as noise). In the spread-spectrum technique, sender transmits a narrowband signal over a much larger bandwidth, such that the signal energy present in any single frequency bin is undetectable. Similarly, the watermark is spread over many frequency bins so that the energy in any one bin is very small and certainly undetectable. Nevertheless, since the watermark verification process is aware of the location and content of the watermark, it is possible to concentrate several weak signals into a single output signal having a high signal-to-noise ratio (SNR) [9]. However, to destroy such a watermark it would require noise of high amplitude which should be added to all frequency bins. Spreading the watermark throughout the spectrum of an image ensures a large measure of security against unintentional or intentional attack. First, the watermark is not present at a fixed location and second the selection of suitable frequency regions ensures that very small energy is present in any single coefficient. A watermark that is well placed in the transform domain of an image will be practically impossible to observe.

3.2.4 Patchwork Technique

Initially, the patchwork technique was proposed by Bender et al. [10] in 1995. This technique is a statistical process based on a pseudorandom in which patchwork imperceptibly embeds in a cover image a specific statistic, one that has a Gaussian distribution [1]. In the embedding process of the patchwork technique, the owner chooses n-pixel pairs pseudo randomly according to a secret key and modifies the luminance values of the n-pairs of pixels. If the luminance values are x_i and y_i, the modified luminance values are determine by adding '1' to all values of x_i and sub-tract '*1*' to all values of y_i i.e. $\bar{x}_i = x_i + 1$ and $\bar{y}_i = y_i - 1$. The same secret key will be use in the extraction process of the technique (which is based on statistical assumption) and determine the sum $(S) = \sum_{n}^{i=1} \bar{x}_i - \bar{y}_i$. If sum (S) = 2n; the cover image actually contained the watermark, otherwise it should be nearly/approximately zero. In [11, 12], the robustness performance of the patchwork technique is improved in which the cover image hide a watermark longer than one bit.

3.3   Transform Domain Techniques

The spatial domain techniques are easy ways to embed secret information, but these techniques are highly vulnerable to even small cover modifications [13]. Anyone can simply apply signal processing techniques in order to destroy entire secret information. In many cases even small changes resulting out of lossy compression systems lead to total information loss. However, the embedding of information in transform domain provides greater robustness of watermarked data. The transform domain techniques hide secret information in significant areas of the cover image which makes them highly robust to signal processing attacks than the spatial domain techniques. The important transform domain techniques are presented in the next sub-sections.

3.3.1   Discrete Wavelet Transform (DWT)

The wavelet is a finite energy function i.e. $\psi \in L^2$ (finite energy function) with zero mean and is normalized ($\|\psi\| = 1$) [14]. A family of wavelets can be obtained by scaling ψ by s and translating it by u.

$$\psi_{u,s}(t) = s^{-1/2} \psi\left(\frac{t-u}{s}\right) \qquad (3.2)$$

The continuous wavelet transform (CWT) of finite energy which is the sum over all time of scaled and shifted versions of the mother wavelet ψ for a 1-D signal $f(t)$ is given by:

$$f(u,s) = \int_{\infty}^{-\infty} (t) s^{-\frac{1}{2}} \psi'\left(\frac{t-u}{s}\right) dt \qquad (3.3)$$

where $\psi'(.)$ is the complex conjugate of $\psi(.)$. Equation (3.3) can be viewed as convolution of the signal with dilated band-pass filters. A continuous signal can be sampled so that a value is recorded after a discrete time interval. If the sampling of signal is carried out at the Nyquist rate, no information would be lost. After sampling the discrete wavelet series could be used. However, this can still be very slow to compute. The reason is that the information available through evaluation of wavelet series is still highly redundant and the solution requires a large amount of computation time. In order to make the wavelet computationally simple, a discrete algorithm is needed. The DWT provides sufficient information both for analysis and synthesis of the original signal with a significant reduction in the computation time. In addition, DWT is considerably easier to implement in comparison to the continuous wavelet transform (CWT). DWT is one of the well-known techniques for sub-band image coding which has considerable attention in various signal processing applications, including image watermarking. The main idea behind DWT results from the multi-resolution analysis, which involves decomposition of an image in frequency channels of constant bandwidth on a logarithmic scale [15]. It has the advantages such as similarity of the data structure with respect to the resolution and available decomposition at any level [16]. If x and y are the integer values, the DWT is defined as [17]:

$$S_{x,y} = \int_{\infty}^{-\infty} \psi'_{x,y}(t)s(t)dt, \qquad (3.4)$$

The inverse of the DWT is defined as:

$$s(t) = C_{\psi} \sum_{x} \sum_{y} S_{x,y} \psi_{x,y}(t) \qquad (3.5)$$

where s(t) is the original signal, C_{ψ} is a constant value for normalization. $\psi_{x,y}(t)$ provides sampling points on the scale-time plane—linear and logarithmic sampling in the time and scale direction, respectively.

DWT separates an image into a set of four non-overlapping multi-resolution sub-bands denoted as lower resolution approximation image (LL) as well as horizontal (HL), vertical (LH) and diagonal (HH) detail components [18]. The process can then be repeated to compute multiple scale wavelet decomposition. Since the human eyes are much more sensitive to the low-frequency part (LL sub-band), the watermark can be embedded into the other three sub-bands (HL, LH and HH sub-band) to maintain better image quality. Figure 3.1 shows the pyramid structure of three levels DWT sub-band. It is evident that the energy of an image is concentrated in the high decomposition levels corresponding to the perceptually significant low frequency coefficients. The low decomposition levels accumulate a minor energy proportion, thus being vulnerable to image alterations. Therefore, the watermarks containing crucial medical information such as doctor's reference, patient identification code, image codes etc. and requiring significantly great robustness are embedded in higher level sub-bands [19]. Figure 3.2 shows the four levels DWT sub-band decomposition of CT test image. The main advantages of wavelet transform domain for watermarking applications are [20–22]:

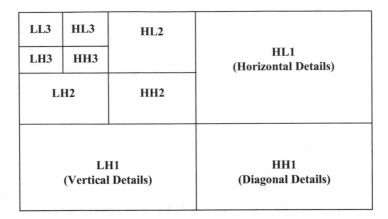

LL3	HL3	HL2	HL1 (Horizontal Details)
LH3	HH3		
LH2		HH2	
LH1 (Vertical Details)			HH1 (Diagonal Details)

Fig. 3.1 Pyramid structure of three levels DWT

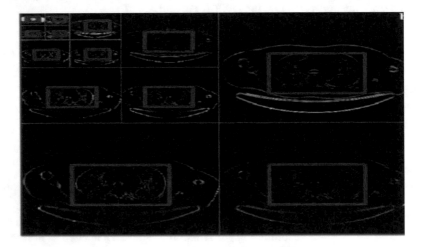

Fig. 3.2 Four level sub-band decomposition of CT test image [19]

1. Space frequency localization: Used for the analysis of edges and textured areas as it provides good space frequency localization.
2. Multi-resolution representation: The multi-resolution property of the wavelet transform can be used to exploit the fact that the response of the human eye is different to high and low frequency components of an image.
3. Multi-scale analysis: Wavelets have non-uniform frequency spectra which facilitate multi-scale analysis.
4. Adaptability: Flexible and easily adaptable to a given set of images or application.
5. Linear complexity: Linear computational complexity of O(n) is present for wavelet transform
6. DWT can be applied to entire image without imposing block structure as used by DCT, thereby reducing blocking artifact.

There are a wide variety of popular wavelet algorithms, including Daubechies wavelets, Mexican Hat wavelets and Morlet wavelets [23]. These wavelet algorithms have advantage of better resolution for smoothly changing time series. However, they have the disadvantage of being more computationally complex than the Haar wavelets. In addition, the Haar wavelet transform is fast, memory efficient and exactly reversible without the edge effects that are present in other wavelet transforms.

As discussed above, the DWT offer various important properties for medical image watermarking. However, it suffers from poor directional information. Do and Vetterli [24] proposed a directional transform called contourlet transform, which have the properties of multi-resolution, localization, critical sampling, rich directionality using directional filter bank and anisotropy. The contourlet transform can be seen as a discrete form of a particular curvelet transform, which is also a popular multi-scale directional transform [25]. However, the curvelets transform have better directional geometry/features than contourlet.

3.3.2 Discrete Cosine Transform (DCT)

The discrete cosine transform (DCT) works by separating image into parts of different frequencies, low, high and middle frequency coefficients [26–28], makes it much easier to embed the watermark information into middle frequency band that provide an additional resistance to the lossy compression techniques, while avoiding significant modification of the cover image. The DCT has a very good energy compaction property. Figure 3.3 show the different frequencies of an *8x8* DCT block.

The F_L is used to denote the lowest frequency components of the block, while F_H is used to denote the higher frequency components. F_M is chosen as the embedding region so as to provide additional resistance to lossy compression techniques, while avoiding significant modification of the cover image. For the input image, I, of size N x N the DCT coefficients for the transformed output image, D, are computed

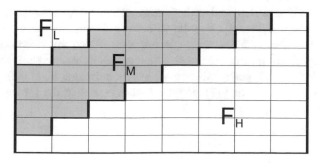

Fig. 3.3 Definition of DCT regions [2]

using Eq. (3.6). The intensity of image is denoted as I (x, y), where the pixel in row x and column y of the image. The DCT coefficient is denoted as D (i, j) where i and j represent the row and column of the DCT matrix.

$$D(i,j) = \frac{1}{\sqrt{2N}} C(i)C(j) \sum_{N-1}^{x=0} \sum_{N-1}^{y=0} I(x,y) \cos\frac{(2x+1)i\pi}{2N} \cos\frac{(2y+1)i\pi}{2N} \quad (3.6)$$

$$C(i), C(j) = \frac{1}{\sqrt{2}} \, for \, i, j = 0$$

$$C(i), C(j) = 1 \, for \, i, j > 0$$

The DCT matrix can be define by using Eq. (3.6):

3.3.3   Singular Value Decomposition (SVD)

The singular value decomposition of a rectangular matrix A is as follows [29]:

$$A = USV^T \quad (3.7)$$

where A is an $M \times N$ matrix, U and V are the orthonormal matrices. S is a diagonal matrix which consists of singular values of A. The singular values appear in the descending order ($s_1 \geq s_2 \geq s_3 \geq \ldots \geq s_n \geq 0$) along with the main diagonal of S. However, these singular values have been obtained by taking the square root of the Eigen values of AA^T and A^TA. These singular values are unique, however the matrices U and V are not unique. The relation between SVD and eigenvalues are:

$$A = USV^T$$

Now $AA^T = USV^T(USV^T)^T = US^2U^T$
Also, $A^T = (USV^T)^TUSV^T = VS^2V^T$

Thus, U and V are calculated as the eigenvectors of AA^T and A^TA, respectively. If the matrix A is real, then the singular values are always real numbers, and U and V are also real. The SVD has two main properties from the viewpoint of image processing applications are: (1) the singular values of an image have very good stability. When a small perturbation is added to an image, its singular values do not change significantly, and (2) singular values represent the intrinsic algebraic image properties [16].

3.3.4 Discrete Fourier Transform (DFT)

The discrete Fourier transform (DFT) was immediately considered in the field of watermarking in order to offer the possibility of controlling the frequencies of the cover data. It is helpful to select the adequate parts of the image for embedding the watermark in order to obtain the optimize trade-off between imperceptibility and robustness. Two major advantages of DFT over the spatial domain techniques are [30]: (1) translation invariant and rotation resistant, which provides strong robustness against geometric attacks, and (2) the watermark information is spread over the entire image, which enables the implementation of stronger watermarks with less perceptual impact. On other hand, fast Fourier transform (FFT) methods introduce round-off errors, which may lead to loss of quality and errors in watermark extraction, as reported in [31]. Unfortunately, this limitation is more important for hidden communication [30]. To determine the DFT of an image F (m, n) of size $M \times N$ image is G (k, l) whereas:

$$G(k,l) = \frac{1}{M \times N} \sum_{M-1}^{m=0} \sum_{N-1}^{n=0} F(m,n) e^{-j2\pi\left[\frac{km}{M}+\frac{nl}{N}\right]} \qquad (3.8)$$

The inverse of DFT is defined as

$$F(m,n) = \sum_{M-1}^{k=0} \sum_{N-1}^{l=0} G(k,l) e^{j2\pi\left[\frac{mk}{M}+\frac{nl}{N}\right]} \qquad (3.9)$$

The DFT is computationally efficient however, the complexity and poor energy compaction properties is the major disadvantages of the DFT.

3.4 Performance Measures

The performance of a medical image watermarking algorithms is mainly evaluated on the basis of its *imperceptibility* and *robustness*.

3.4.1 Mean Square Error (MSE)

The MSE contains the cumulative squared error between original and watermarked image [32]. A lower value of MSE indicates that the visual quality of the image will be near to original one. The MSE can be defined as:

$$MSE = \frac{1}{X \times Y} \sum_{i=1}^{X} \sum_{i=1}^{Y} \left(I_{ij} - W_{ij} \right)^2 \tag{3.10}$$

where I_{ij} is a pixel of the original image of size $X \times Y$ and W_{ij} is a pixel of the watermarked image of size $X \times Y$.

3.4.2   Peak Signal-to-Noise Ratio (PSNR)

The *imperceptibility* is measured by the parameter Peak Signal to Noise Ratio (PSNR). A larger PSNR indicates that the watermarked image more closely resembles the original image which conveys the meaning that the watermark is more imperceptible. In general, the watermarked image with PSNR value greater than 28 dB is acceptable [33]. The PSNR is defined as:

$$PSNR = 10 \log \frac{(255)^2}{MSE} \tag{3.11}$$

3.4.3   Weighted Peak Signal to Noise Ratio (WPSNR)

The WPSNR is modified version of the PSNR [33]. The WPSNR defined as:

$$WPSNR = 10 \log_{10} \frac{(255)^2}{NVF \times MSE} \tag{3.12}$$

where the *noise visibility function (NVF)* depends on a texture masking function. Its values range from zero (for extremely textured areas) to one (for smooth areas of an image).

3.4.4   Universal Image Quality Index

Wang and Bovik [34] define a universal image quality index which is a significant performance parameter to determine image distortion as a function of loss of correlation, luminance and contrast distortion. The Universal image quality index parameter determines the image distortion significantly better than the other image distortion metrics like MSE. Suppose X is the original image and Y is possibly distorted image whereas, X=$\{x_i, i = 1, 2, 3, \ldots \ldots \ldots N\}$ and Y=$\{y_i, i = 1, 2, 3, \ldots \ldots \ldots N\}$. The universal image quality index is defined as:

$$Q = \frac{4\sigma_{xy}\overline{x}\overline{y}}{\left(\sigma_x^2 + \sigma_y^2\right)\left(\overline{x}^2 + \overline{y}^2\right)} \tag{3.13}$$

where $\overline{x} = \dfrac{1}{N}\sum_{N}^{i=1} x_i$ and $\overline{y} = \dfrac{1}{N}\sum_{N}^{i=1} y_i$

$$\sigma_x^2 = \frac{1}{N-1}\sum_{N}^{i=1}(x_i - \overline{x})^2, \ \sigma_y^2 = \frac{1}{N-1}\sum_{N}^{i=1}(y_i - \overline{y})^2, \ \sigma_{xy} = \frac{1}{N-1}\sum_{N}^{i=1}(x_i - \overline{x})(y_i - \overline{y})$$

The term 'Q' can also define the product of three components:

$$Q = \left\{ \text{loss of correlation} \left(\frac{\sigma_{xy}}{\sigma_x \sigma_y}\right) \cdot \text{luminance distortion} \left(\frac{2\overline{x}\overline{y}}{(\overline{x})^2 + (\overline{y})^2}\right) \cdot \text{contrast distortion} \left(\frac{2\sigma_x \sigma_y}{\sigma_x^2 + \sigma_y^2}\right) \right\}$$

These components define as:

1. The loss of correlation define the linear correlation between x and y with dynamic range [−1, 1].
2. The luminance distortion is to determine the how close the mean luminance between x and y with range of [0, 1].
3. The contrast distortion is to determine the contrast similarities between images with range of [0, 1].

3.4.5 Structural Similarity Index Measure (SSIM)

The SSIM [33] can be defined as:

$$SSIM(x,y) = f\big(l(x,y),c(x,y),s(x,y)\big) \tag{3.14}$$

where $l(x, y)$, $c(x, y)$ and $s(x, y)$ are luminance measurement, contrast measurement and structure measurement respectively are the important property of an image.

3.4.6 Normalized Correlation (NC)

The *robustness* of a watermarking algorithm is measured in terms of Normalized Correlation (NC) and bit error rate (BER). NC value measures the similarity and differences between the original watermark and extracted watermark. Its value is generally 0–1. However, ideally it should be 1 but the value 0.7 is acceptable [35].

$$NC = \sum_{X}^{i=1} \sum_{Y}^{j=1} \left(W_{\text{original}_{ij}} \times W_{\text{recovered}_{ij}} \right) / \sum_{X}^{i=1} \sum_{Y}^{j=1} W_{\text{original}_{ij}}^{2} \qquad (3.15)$$

where $W_{\text{original}_{ij}}$ is a pixel of the original/hidden watermark of size $X \times Y$ and $W_{\text{recovered}_{ij}}$ is a pixel of the recovered watermark of size $X \times Y$.

3.4.7 Bit Error Rate (BER)

The BER is defined as the ratio of the number of incorrectly decoded bits and total number of bits [35]. This parameter is suitable for random binary sequence watermark. Ideally BER value should be equal to 0.

$$BER = \left(\text{Number of incorrectly decoded bits} \right) / \left(\text{Total number of bits} \right) \qquad (3.16)$$

3.5 Digital Watermarking Attacks and Benchmark Tools

In recent years, digital image watermarking most widely used techniques for prevention of copyright violation, ownership identification, and identity theft. However, robustness/security of the watermark in a medical application have been challenging issues due to attempts of malicious attacks/hacking of open channel information [36]. The purpose behind attacks can be to alter, modify, or even delete the document watermark from its cover data to illegally claim ownership or preventing the information transfer to intended recipients.

3.5.1 Watermarking Attacks

There are several kinds of malicious attacks, which result in a partial or even total destruction of the embed identification key and for which more advanced watermarking scheme should employed [33, 36–39]. Figure 3.4 shows the possible attacks in watermarking systems. The important attacks are discussed below:

1. *Active/Removal Attacks*: In this type of attack, the hacker tries deliberately to remove the watermark or simply make it undetectable. They are aimed at distorting a hidden watermark beyond recognition. The active attacks include

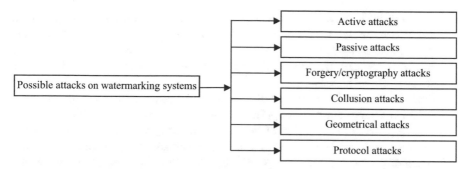

Fig. 3.4 Classification of possible attacks in digital watermarking

de-noising, lossy compression, quantization, re-modulation, collusion and averaging attacks. This is a big issue in copyright protection, fingerprinting or copy control for example.

2. *Passive Attacks*: Hacker tries to determine whether there is a watermark and identify it. However, no damage or removal is done. As the reader should understand, protection against passive attacks is of the utmost importance in covert communications where the simple knowledge of the presence of watermark is often more than one want to grant.

3. *Forgery/Cryptography Attacks*: This is another type of active attacks. In such attacks, the hacker embeds a new, valid watermark rather than removing one. This will help him to manipulate the protected data as he wants and then, re-implant a new given key to replace the destructed one, thus making the corrupted image seems genuine. One of the similar techniques in this category brute force attacks used in cryptography which aim to finds hidden information through an exhaustive search. For these types of attacks, it is very important to use a key of secure length as reported in [36]. The Oracle attack is the same category of the cryptographic attacks in which a non-watermarked image is created when a watermark detector device is available.

4. *Collusion Attacks*: In such attacks, the intention of the hacker is the same as for the active attacks but the approach is slightly different. The attacker uses many instances of the same data, containing each different watermark, to construct a new copy without any watermark. This is a problem in finger printing applications but is not widely spread because the attacker should be able to access several copies of the same data and that the number needed can be very important. Collusion Attacks should be considered because if the attacker has access to more than one copy of watermarked image, the user can predict/remove the watermarked data by colluding them given key to replace the destructed one, thus making the corrupted image seem genuine.

5. *Geometrical Attacks*: The aim of geometrical attacks is to alter/distort the hidden watermark through spatial or temporal alterations of the stego data. Due to this type of active attack, the watermark detector loses the synchronization with the hidden watermark. Unzign and Stirmark are the popular integrated software for the geometrical attacks.
6. *Protocol Attacks*: The objective of these types of passive attacks is to attack the concept of the watermarking application instead of destroying the hidden watermark or disable the detection of the hidden watermark through local or global data manipulation. The concept of first protocol attacks was given in. The another group of protocol attacks is copy attack in which copy a watermark from one image to another image without knowledge of the key used for the watermark embedding to create ambiguity with respect to the real ownership of data.

3.5.2   Benchmark Tools for Image Watermarking

Benchmarking of digital watermarking algorithms is the process of evaluating and comparing their performance under a fair and normally (semi-)automated environment [40]. The important benchmarking tools for watermarking are StirMark [41–43], CheckMark [44, 45], Optimark [46, 47] and Certimark [48].

Stir-Mark benchmark is a most popular and excellent software tool which is used to determine the robustness performance of the different watermarking systems. This tool simulates various common attacks to image watermarking algorithms which do not survive Stir-Mark attacks should be insecure, as reported in [40]. Unfortunately, it does not properly model the watermarking process and therefore is limited in its potential for impairing sophisticated image watermarking techniques. Further, the Stir-Mark benchmark tool is heavily weighted towards geometric transformations, which do not take into account prior information about the watermark [37]. Therefore, another benchmark tool 'Checkmark' was developed by Pereira et al. [45]. This tool is basically improved version of Stirmark with following major changes [40]:

1. The Checkmark tool includes Wiener filtering, soft shrinkage, hard thresholding, Copy, Template removal and JPEG 2000 as new attacks,
2. Weighted PSNR and Watson's metric are included instead of just PSNT to determine the visual quality of the image, and
3. The checkmark tool is implemented in MATLAB; however the Stirmark is implemented in C++.

Another important benchmark tools are Optimark [46, 47] which is a benchmarking software package for image watermarking algorithms providing a graphical user interface (GUI) implemented in C/C++. To use optimark determine the performance of watermarking algorithm, users may select a set of test images, define different watermark embedding keys and messages for multiple trials of the watermarking detector and decoder, and select a set of attacks among different types of attacks and its combinations. Further, it allows the assessment of several statistical characteristics of an image watermarking algorithm. The Certimark benchmark tool was developed by EU-funded research project in 2000–2002 [40]. Objective of this tool is to design a benchmarking collection module which allows users to assess the suitability and to set application scenarios for their needs, and to set up a standard certification process for watermarking technologies [48]. Unfortunately, source codes are not publicly available for this tool. In addition to that some researcher proposed benchmark tool based on web system [49–53], mesh benchmark [54] and OR-benchmark tool [40] for evaluating the performance of watermarking algorithms. The brief comparison of the above benchmarking tool has been discussed detail in [40].

3.6 Summary

In this chapter, the authors have presented important spatial and transform domain techniques followed by the major performance parameters for medical as well as digital image watermarking. It includes peak signal to noise ratio (PSNR), weighted peak signal to noise ratio (WPSNR), Universal image quality index, Structural similarity index measure (SSIM), normalized correlation (NC), and bit error rate (BER). Further, we have presented a brief description of different types of attack and important benchmarking tools along with their performance comparison for digital image watermarking. We have noticed that the performance of efficient and robust watermarking algorithm (s) are highly depends on the types of attacks. In addition, the developments of the efficient benchmarking tools are necessary to require with rich features in near future. However, the available benchmarking tools are not sufficient.

References

1. D. Arya, A survey of frequency and wavelet domain digital watermarking techniques. Int. J. Sci. Eng. Res. **1**(2), 1–4 (2010)
2. C. Shoemaker, *Hidden Bits: A Survey of Techniques for Digital Watermarking*, Independent Study (Spring, 2002)
3. O. Bruyndonckx, J.J. Quisquater, B. Macq, Spatial method for copyright labeling of digital images, in Proceeding of IEEE Workshop on Nonlinear Signal and Image Processing, Neos Marmaras, Greece, pp. 456–459, 1995
4. N. Nikolaidis, I. Pitas, Robust image watermarking in the spatial domain. Signal Process. **66**(3), 385–403 (1998)
5. A.K. Singh, N. Sharma, M. Dave, A. Mohan, A novel technique for digital image watermarking in spatial domain, in Proceeding of 2nd International Conference on Parallel Distributed and Grid Computing, Jaypee University of Information Technology, Waknaghat, Solan, Himachal Pradesh, India, pp. 497–501, 2012

6. G. Langelaar, I. Setyawan, R. Lagendijk, Watermarking digital image and video data: a state-of-art overview. IEEE Signal Process. Mag. **17**(5), 20–46 (2000)
7. A.K. Parthasarathy, S. Kak, An improved method of content based image watermarking. IEEE Trans. Broadcast. **53**(2), 468–479 (2007)
8. I.J. Cox, J. Kilian, F.T. Leighton, T. Shamoon, Secure spread spectrum watermarking for multimedia. IEEE Trans. Image Process. **6**(12), 1673–1687 (1997)
9. B. Kumar, H.V. Singh, S.P. Singh, A. Mohan, Secure spread-spectrum watermarking for tele-medicine applications. J. Inf. Secur. **2**(2), 91–98 (2011)
10. W. Bender, D. Gruhl, N. Morimoto, Techniques for data hiding, in Proceedings of the SPIE 2420, Storage and Retrieval for Image and Video Databases III, pp. 164–173, 1995
11. G.C. Langelaar, J.C.A. Van der Lubbe, R.L. Lagendijk, Robust labeling methods for copy protection of images, in Proceedings of SPIE 3022, Storage and Retrieval for Image and Video Databases V, pp. 298–309, 1997
12. I. Pitas, T.H. Kaskalis, Applying signatures on digital images, in IEEE Workshop on Nonlinear Signal and Image Processing, Thessaloniki, Greece, pp. 460–463, 1995
13. K.T. Lin, Digital image hiding in an image using n-graylevel encoding, in Proceeding of 1st International Conference on Information Science and Engineering, IEEE Computer Society, Washington, DC, USA, pp. 1720–1724, 2009
14. R. Chellappa, S. Theodoridis, *Academic Press Library in Signal Processing: Signal Processing Theory and Machine Learning*, vol 1 (Elsevier, 2014)
15. A.K. Singh, M. Dave, A. Mohan, Hybrid technique for robust and imperceptible multiple watermarking using medical images. J. Multimedia Tools Appl. **75**(14), 8381–8401 (2015). doi:10.1007/s11042-015-2754-7
16. C.-C. Lai, C.-C. Tsai, Digital image watermarking using discrete wavelet transform and singular value decomposition. IEEE Trans. Instrum. Meas. **59**(11), 3060–3063 (2010)
17. D.T.L. Lee, A. Yamamoto, Wavelet analysis: theory and applications. Hewlett-Packard J. **5**, 44–52 (1994)
18. M.K. Gupta, S. Tiwari, Performance evaluation of conventional and wavelet based OFDM system. AEU—Int. J. Electron. Commun. **67**(4), 348–354 (2013)
19. A. Giakoumaki, S. Pavlopoulos, D. Koutsouris, Secure and efficient health data management through multiple watermarking on medical images. Med. Biol. Eng. Comput. **44**(8), 619–631 (2006)
20. P. Meerwald, A. Uhl, Survey of wavelet-domain watermarking algorithms, in Proceedings of the SPIE Security and Watermarking of Multimedia Contents III, San Jose, pp. 505–516, 2001
21. G. Carl, R.R. Brooks, S. Rai, Wavelet based denial-of-service detection. Comput. Security **25**(8), 600–615 (2006)
22. A.H. Paquet, R.K. Ward, Wavelet-based digital watermarking for authentication, in Proceedings of the IEEE Canadian Conference on Electrical and Computer Engineering, Winnipeg, pp. 879–884, 2002
23. X.-y. Chen, Y.-y. Zhan, Multi-scale anomaly detection algorithm based on infrequent pattern of time series. J. Comput. Appl. Math. **214**(1), 227–237 (2008)
24. M. Do, M. Vetterli, The contourlet transform: an efficient directional multiresolution image representation. IEEE Trans. Image Process. **14**(12), 2091–2106 (2005)
25. G. Jianwei Ma, Plonka, The curvelet transform. IEEE Signal Process. Mag. **27**(2), 118–133 (2010)
26. A. Al-Haj, Combined DWT–DCT digital image watermarking. J. Comput. Sci. **3**(9), 740–746 (2007)
27. J.R. Hernandez, M. Amado, F. Perez-Gonzalez, DCT-Domain watermarking techniques for still images: detector performance analysis and a new structure. IEEE Trans. Image Process. **9**(1), 55–68 (2000)
28. K. Viswanath, J. Mukherjee, P.K. Biswas, Image filtering in the block DCT domain using symmetric convolution. J. Vis. Commun. Image Represent. **22**(2), 141–152 (2011)

29. D. Kalman, A singularly valuable decomposition: the SVD of a matrix, The American University, February 13, 2002
30. A. Poljicak, L. Mandic, D. Agic, Discrete Fourier transform–based watermarking method with an optimal implementation radius. J. Electron. Imaging **20**(3), 033008 (2011)
31. A. Cheddad, J. Condell, K. Curran, M. Kevitt, Digital image steganography: survey and analysis of current methods. Signal Process. **90**, 727–752 (2010)
32. Z. Wang, A.C. Bovik, Mean squared error: love it or leave it? A new look at signal fidelity measures. IEEE Signal Process. Mag. **26**, 98–117 (2009)
33. A.K. Singh, B. Kumar, M. Dave, S.P. Ghrera, A. Mohan, Digital image watermarking: techniques and emerging applications, in *Handbook of Research on Modern Cryptographic Solutions for Computer and Cyber Security*, (IGI Global, Hershey, 2016), pp. 246–272
34. Z. Wang, A.C. Bovik, A universal image quality index. IEEE Signal Process. Lett. **9**(3), 81–84 (2002)
35. A.K. Singh, Improved hybrid technique for robust and imperceptible multiple watermarking using medical images. Multimedia Tools Appl. **76**(6), 8881–8900 (2017)
36. S. Voloshynovskiy, S. Pereira, V. Iquise, T. Pun, Attack modelling: towards a second generation watermarking benchmark. Signal Process. **81**(6), 1177–1214 (2001)
37. S. Voloshynovskiy, S. Pereira, T. Pun, J.J. Eggers, J.K. Su, Attacks on digital watermarks: classification, estimation-based attacks and benchmarks. IEEE Commun. Mag. **39**, 118–126 (2001)
38. C. Song, S. Sudirman, M. Merabti, D. Llewellyn-Jones, Analysis of digital image watermark attacks, in 7th IEEE Consumer Communications and Networking Conference, Las Vegas, Nevada, USA, pp. 941–945, January 09–12, 2010
39. H. Nyeem, W. Boles, C. Boyd, Digital image watermarking: its formal model, fundamental properties and possible attacks. EURASIP J. Adv. Signal Process. **135**, 1–22 (2014)
40. H. Wang, A.T.S. Ho, S. Li, OR-benchmark: an open and reconfigurable digital watermarking benchmarking framework, June 02, 2015
41. F.A.P. Petitcolas, M. Steinebach, F. Raynal, J. Dittman, C. Fontaine, N. Fates, in *A Public Automated Web-Based Evaluation Service for Watermarking Schemes: Stir Mark Benchmark*, ed. by P.W. Wong, E.J. Delp. Proceedings of the SPIE/IS&T Conference on Security and Watermarking of Multimedia Contents, San Jose, CA, vol. 4314, 2001
42. F.A.P. Petitcolas, R.J. Anderson, M.G. Kuhn, Attacks on copyright marking systems, in *Information Hiding, Second International Workshop*, ed. by D. Aucsmith (Ed), (Springer-Verlag, Portland, OR, 1998), pp. 219–239
43. F.A.P. Petitcolas, Watermarking schemes evaluation. IEEE Signal Process. Mag. **17**(5), 58–64 (2000)
44. http://watermarking.unige.ch/Checkmark/
45. S. Pereira, S. Voloshynovskiy, M. Madueño, S. Marchand-Maillet, T. Pun, Second generation benchmarking and application oriented evaluation, in Information Hiding Workshop, Pittsburgh, PA, 2001
46. V. Solachidis, A. Tefas, N. Nikolaidis, S. Tsekeridou, A. Nikolaidis, P. Pitas, A benchmarking protocol for watermarking methods, in Proceedings of the IEEE International Conference on Image Processing, vol. 3, Thessaloniki, Greece, pp. 1023–1026, 2001
47. http://poseidon.csd.auth.gr/optimark/
48. J.C. Vorbruggen, F. Cayre, The Certimark benchmark: architecture and future perspectives, in Proceedings of 2002 IEEE International Conference on Multimedia and Expo (ICME 2002), vol. 2, pp. 485–488, 2002
49. H.C. Kim, H. Ogunleye, O. Guitart, E.J. Delp, The watermark evaluation test bed (WET). Proc. SPIE **5306**, 236–247 (2004)
50. H.C. Kim, E.T. Lin, O. Guitart, E.J.D. III, Further progress in watermark evaluation test bed (WET). Proc. SPIE **5681**, 241–251 (2005)
51. O. Guitart, H. C. Kim, and E. J. D. III, "The watermark evaluation testbed (WET): new functionalities," in Proc. SPIE, vol. 6072. 2006, art. no. 607210.

52. S. Lugan, B. Macq, Thread-based benchmarking deployment. Proc. SPIE **5306**, 248–255 (2004)
53. B. Michiels, B. Macq, Benchmarking image watermarking algorithms with open water-mark, in Proceedings of 14th European Signal Processing Conference, Florence, Italy, pp. 1–5, 2006
54. K. Wang, G. Lavoue, F. Denis, A. Baskurt, X. He, A benchmark for 3D mesh watermarking, in Proceedings of 2010 IEEE International Conference on Shape Modeling and Applications (SMI 2010), pp. 231–235, 2010

Chapter 4
Robust and Imperceptible Hybrid Watermarking Techniques for Medical Images

Amit Kumar Singh, Basant Kumar, Ghanshyam Singh, and Anand Mohan

4.1 Introduction

The information and communication technology (ICT) has eased the duplication, manipulation and distribution of digital data in recent times which has resulted in the demand for safe ownership of digital images and the potential solution to the problem of copyright protection and content authentication is the digital watermarking. However, a single watermarking method can only serve for a limited number of purposes. As reported earlier, the DWT, DCT and SVD are popular transform domain techniques used for watermarking. To overcome the limitations of single watermarking technique, a hybrid watermarking method is a superior choice, as reported in various literatures [1–21]. Consequently, several hybrid watermarking techniques which have been combined DWT, DCT and SVD methods as reported in [22–26].

A.K. Singh (✉)
Department of Computer Science & Engineering, Jaypee University of Information
Technology, Waknaghat, Solan, India
e-mail: amit_245singh@yahoo.com

B. Kumar
Department of Electronics and Communication Engineering, Motilal Nehru National
Institute of Technology, Allahabad, India
e-mail: singhbasant@yahoo.com

G. Singh
Department of Electronics and Communication Engineering, Jaypee University
of Information Technology, Waknaghat, Solan, India
e-mail: drghanshyam.singh@yahoo.com

A. Mohan
Department of Electronics Engineering, Indian Institute of Technology (BHU),
Varanasi, India
e-mail: profanandmohan@gmail.com

© Springer International Publishing AG 2017
A.K. Singh et al. (eds.), *Medical Image Watermarking*, Multimedia Systems
and Applications, DOI 10.1007/978-3-319-57699-2_4

The rest of the chapter is organized as follows. The related and recent state-of-the-art techniques are provided in Sect. 4.2. Section 4.3 provides the main contribution of the proposed work. The proposed technique is detailed in Sect. 4.4. Encryption and decryption processes are presented in Sect. 4.5. The experimental results and brief analysis of the work is reported in Sect. 4.6. Next, our summary of the chapter is presented in Sect. 4.7.

4.2 Related Work

Various recent hybrid watermarking techniques are presented as follows. Singh et al. [22] proposed a hybrid algorithm for image watermarking based on DWT, DCT, and SVD by first decomposing the host and watermark image into first level DWT. This is followed by transforming both the high frequency band (HH) of the cover image and watermark image using DCT and SVD. The 'S' vector of watermark information is embedded in the S component of the host image. The performance of Haar, Daubechies2, Biorthogonal1.1, and Coiflet1 filters against different signal processing attacks have been evaluated and compared. Khan et al. [23] proposed a hybrid method for image watermarking using DWT, DCT and SVD in a zig-zag order. The proposed method has been extensively tested against known attacks and has been found to give superior performance for robustness and imperceptibility as compared to the existing methods based on DCT–SVD or DWT only. Srivastva and Saxena [24] proposed a semi-blind image watermarking method based on DWT, DCT and SVD, in which the host and the watermark images are decomposed into first level DWT and then the watermark is transformed by DCT and SVD before embedding it into middle frequency band of the cover image. The method is robust against various attacks. Harish et al. [25] also developed a hybrid method based on DWT, DCT and SVD. This embedding process uses modification of the singular values of the DCT coefficients of the cover image with the singular values of the watermark image. The proposed method is shown to be robust against various attacks. Rosiyadi et al. [27] proposed a hybrid watermarking method based on DCT and SVD for the copyright protection. In this embedding process, DCT is applied on the host image using the zig-zag space-filling curve (SFC) for the DCT coefficients and subsequently the SVD is applied on the DCT coefficients. Finally, the host image is modified by the left singular vectors and the singular values of the DCT coefficients to embed the watermark image. In this method, genetic algorithm (GA) based technique is used for the optimization scaling factor of the watermark image. The experimental results have shown that the proposed method is robust against several kinds of attacks. The comparison between the method based on DCT and SVD using GA and the hybrid method based on DCT-SVD has been presented by Rosiyadi et al. in [28]. It is shown that the robustness of extracted watermark and the visual quality of the watermarked image of the method using GA technique is better than that of the hybrid method.

Horng et al. [29] proposed a blind watermarking method based on DCT, SVD and GA. It is shown that this method is robust and offers high imperceptibility against several known attacks. Horng et al. [30] proposed an adaptive watermarking method based on DCT, SVD and GA. In this embedding process, the host image luminance masking is used and the mask of each sub-band area is transformed into frequency domain. Subsequently, the watermark image is embedded by modifying the singular values of DCT-transformed host image with singular values of mask coefficients of host image and the control parameter of DCT-transformed watermark image using GA. It is shown that this method is robust against several known attacks. Ali et al. [31] proposed a watermarking scheme based on Differential Evolution using DWT and SVD. In the embedding process, the singular vector of selected DWT sub-band of the cover is modified with binary watermark image. The proposed method claimed that it offer the solution for false positive problem as suffer by SVD.

In [32], the authors present a multiple watermarking method using combination of DWT and SVD. Further, the method enhanced the security and robustness of the watermark information, encryption and Reed-Solomon ECC is applied to the watermark before embedding into the cover medical image. The method is robust for different attacks including the Checkmark attacks. In [33], the authors presents a multiple watermarking technique based on discrete wavelet transforms (DWT), discrete cosine transform (DCT) and singular value decomposition (SVD) for healthcare applications. Further, the robustness and security of the considered image watermark is enhanced by using Back Propagation Neural Network (BPNN) and Arnold transform, respectively. Moreover, two different text watermarks called symptom and signature are also encoded by lossless compression technique and error correction code, respectively. The experimental results demonstrated that the method is robust for various attacks. The performance of method is also compared with some recent reported techniques. A region based robust and secure watermarking method is presented by Sharma et al. [34] for medical applications. The method initially uses DWT and DCT to embed multiple watermark information in to the cover medical image. Further, the security of image and text watermark information is enhanced by message-digest (MD5) hash algorithm and Rivest–Shamir–Adleman (RSA) respectively before embedding into the medical cover image. In order to enhance the robustness of text watermark, hamming error correction code is also applied on the encrypted watermark. The experimental results have been shown that the method is robust for important signal processing attacks.

4.3 Main Contribution of the Work

In this chapter, we have proposed a robust hybrid watermarking technique using fusion of DWT, DCT and SVD. The robustness performance of the proposed technique is also tested for known and 'Checkmark' attacks. The technique is found to be robust for all the considered attacks. Moreover, the performance of the proposed algorithm has also been evaluated for multiple watermarking (image and text), which is presented in Sect. 4.6.2. In order to enhance the security of the text watermark, encryption is applied to the text watermark before embedding. The results are obtained by varying the gain factor, size of the text watermark, and cover medical images. The method has been extensively tested and analyzed against known attacks and giving superior performance for robustness, capacity and reduced storage and bandwidth requirements compared to reported techniques suggested by other authors. Further, the robustness and capacity performance of the hybrid multiple watermarking is improved in Sect. 4.6.3.

4.4 Proposed Method

The proposed method for watermarking based on DWT, SVD and DCT increases the robustness without significant degradation of cover image quality against the signal processing attacks. The performance of proposed hybrid method has also been evaluated for multiple watermarks image and text. The technique has four parts, the image watermark embedding and extraction processes, and the text watermark embedding and extraction processes. The method proposed in [35] was modified to embed and extract text watermark. The details of the four algorithms are given in separate subsections:

4.4.1 Embedding Algorithm for Image Watermark

In this algorithm, the considered cover image is decomposed by DWT where the low frequency sub-band is transformed by DCT and SVD. The watermark image is also transformed by DCT and SVD. The singular value of watermark information is embedded in the singular value of the cover image. The detail of embedding algorithm for the image watermark is presented as follows.

start:
STEP 1: Variable Declaration
Barbara Image: cover image
Medical Image (Thorax): watermark image
C_w: read the cover image
W_w: read the watermark image
α : gain factor
DWT, DCT and SVD: Transform Domain Techniques
Wavelet filters: Haar
LL_c , LH_c , HL_c , and HH_c : First level DWT coefficients for cover image
D: DCT coefficients of watermark image
D_c^1 : DCT coefficients matrix for HH_c
U_c and V_c^T : orthonormal matrices for D_c^1
S_c : diagonal matrix for D_c^1
U_w and V_w^T : orthonormal matrices for D

S_w : diagonal matrix for D
W_w^k : modified value of S_c
U_{ww} and V_{ww}^T : orthonormal matrices for W_w^k
S_{ww} : diagonal matrix for W_w^k
W_{modi} : Modified DWT coefficient
W_{idct} : InverseDCT coefficients matrix
W_d : Watermarked Image

STEP 2: Read the Images
C_w ←MRI.bmp (Cover image of size 512 × 512)
W_w ← Thorax.bmp (Watermark image of size 256 × 256)

STEP 3: Perform DWT on Cover and DCT on Watermark image
Apply first level DWT on cover image
$[LL_c , LH_c , HL_c , HH_c]$ ←DWT(C_w, wavelet filter);
D = DCT(W_w);

STEP 4: Choice of sub-bands in Cover and obtain the DCT coefficients for the same HH_C
//Choose sub-band LL_c from cover image
if (DCT on LL_c) **then**
$D_c^1 \leftarrow DCT(LL_c)$;
endif;

STEP 5: Compute the singular values of DCT coefficients for Cover and Watermark image
if (SVD on D_c^1) **then**
$U_c S_c V_c^T \leftarrow SVD\left(D_c^1\right)$
endif;
if (SVD on D)**then**
$U_w S_w V_w^T \leftarrow SVD(D)$
endif;

STEP 6: Image Watermark Embedding
for $\alpha\leftarrow 0.01{:}0.9$
$S_c + \alpha S_w = W_w^k$;
end;

STEP 7: Compute the singular values for W_w^k and obtain the modified DWT coefficients
if (SVD on W_w^k)**then**
$U_{ww} S_{ww} V_{ww}^T \leftarrow SVD\left(W_w^k\right)$
endif;
//modified DWT coefficient
$W_{modi} \leftarrow U_c S_{ww} V_c^T$

Step 8: Obtain the Watermarked Image.
$W_{idct} \leftarrow inverse(W_{modi})$;
//Apply InverseDWT to LL_c , LH_c , HL_c and HH_c with modified coefficient
$W_d \leftarrow$ InverseDWT(W_{idct} , LH_c , HL_c , HH_cwavelet filter);
end:

4.4.2   Extraction Algorithm for Image Watermark

The extraction algorithm of the image watermark is just reverse process of the embedding algorithm. The detail of the extraction algorithm for the image watermark is presented as follows.

start:
STEP 1: Variable Declaration
α : gain factor
LL_c , LH_c , HL_c , HH_c: sub-bands for watermarked image
D_w^* : DCT coefficients matrix for HH_c
U_w^* and V_w^{*T} : orthonormal matrices for D_w^*
S_w^* :: diagonal matrix for D_w^*
S^{*k}:modified values
U_w^{*1} and V_w^{*1T} : orthonormal matrices for S^{*k}
S_w^{*1} : diagonal matrix for S^{*k}
I_{cc}^* : modified DWT coefficients
W_{EW}: Extracted watermark image

STEP 2: Perform DWT on Watermarked image (possibly distorted)
$[LL_c$, LH_c , HL_c , $HH_c] \leftarrow$ DWT (W_d , wavelet filter);

STEP 3: obtain the DCT coefficients for HH_c
if (DCT on LL_c)**then**
$D_w^* \leftarrow$ DCT (LL_c);
endif;

STEP 4: Compute the singular values for D_w^*
$U_w^* S_w^* V_w^{*T} \leftarrow SVD(D_w^*)$
end;

STEP 5: Perform the operation and then apply SVD
for $\alpha = 0.01{:}0.9$
$$S^{*k} = \frac{S_w^* - S_c}{\alpha}$$
end;
$U_w^{*1} S_w^{*1} V_w^{*1T} \leftarrow SVD(S^{*k})$

STEP 6: Compute modified DWT coefficients
$I_{cc}^* \leftarrow U_w S_w^{*1} V_w^T$

STEP 7: Extract the watermark image.
$W_{EW} \leftarrow$ InverseDCT (I_{cc}^*);
end:

4.4.3 Embedding Algorithm for Text Watermark

The embedding algorithm for text watermark is formulated as follows:

start:
STEP 1: Variable Declaration
Medical Image (MRI): cover image
EPR Data: Text watermark
C_w: read the cover image
W_w: read the text watermark
α : gain factor
DWT : discrete wavelet transforms
Wavelet filters: Haar
LL_c , HL_c , LH_c and HH_c : First level DWT coefficients for cover image
LL_{c1} , HL_{c1} , LH_{c1} and HH_{c1}: Second level DWT coefficients for cover image

STEP 2: Read the Images
M_w$\leftarrow$ MRI.bmp (Cover image of size 512 × 512)

STEP 3: Perform DWT on Cover image
//Apply second level DWT on cover image
[LL_c, HL_c, LH_c and HH_c]$\leftarrow$ DWT (M_w, wavelet filter);
[LL_{c1}, HL_{c1}, LH_{c1} and HH_{c1}]$\leftarrow$DWT (HH_c, wavelet filter);

STEP 4: Encrypt the watermark text using equation (4.1)

STEP 5: Convert encrypted watermarking text to Binary bits
// converting text watermark into binary bits
Wtxt $\leftarrow$ binary(Text Watermark));

STEP 6: Replace '(0,1)' by '(-1,1)' in the watermarking bits
// bit stream is transformed into a sequence w(1) w(2)....w(L) by replacing the 0 by
-1 and 1 by 1, L is the length of string
$-1 \leftarrow 0$ *and* $1 \leftarrow 1$;

STEP 8: Embedding the text watermark
// text watermark is embeds into HH_{c1} sub-band
for $\alpha \leftarrow 0.01 : 0.1$
$f(x, y) = f(x, y)(1 + \alpha \times Wb)$; $f(x, y)$ and $f(x, y)$ is DWT coefficients before and after
embedding process

end;
STEP 9: Obtain the Watermarked Image W_d
//Apply Inverse DWT to LL_c , HL_c , LH_c and HH_c with modified and unmodified DWT coefficients
$W_{mg} = inverse\ DWT(LL_{c1}, HL_{c1}, LH_{c1}\ and\ HH_{c1}, wavelet\ filter)$;
$W_d \leftarrow inverse\ DWT(LL_c, HL_c, LH_c\ and\ W_{mg}, wavelet\ filter)$;
end:

4.4.4 *Extraction Algorithm for Text Watermark*

In the watermark extraction procedure, both the received and original image are decomposed into the second levels. It is assumed that the original image is available for extraction process.

start:
STEP 1: Variable Declaration
Medical Image (MRI): cover image
EPR Data : Text Watermark
C_w: read the cover image
α : gain factor
DWT : discrete wavelet transforms
Wavelet filters: Haar
LL_c , HL_c , LH_c and HH_c : First level DWT coefficients for cover image
LL_{c1} , HL_{c1} , LH_{c1} and HH_{c1}: Second level DWT coefficients for cover image

start:
STEP 2: Perform DWT on Watermarked image (possibly distorted)
// original image is also available for extraction process
$[LL_c, HL_c, LH_c\ and\ HH_c, wavelet\ filter] \leftarrow DWT\ (W_d, wavelet\ filter)$;

STEP 3: Watermark extraction
$$W_r b = \frac{\left(f_r'\left(x,y\right) - f\left(x,y\right)\right)}{\alpha f\left(x,y\right)} ; f_r'(x, y)\ are\ \text{the DWT coefficients of the received image.}$$
//finally extracted watermark taken as sign(either positive or negative)
$W_e b \leftarrow positive\ or\ negative\ \text{sign}(W_r b)$;

STEP 4: Convert the watermark bits into text to get the characters

STEP 5: Decrypt the characters by using Equation (4.2) to get the original watermark
end:

4.5   Encryption and Decryption Process for Text Watermark

For providing additional security, text watermark (EPR data) may be encrypted before watermarking. However, the delay encountered during embedding and extraction of the watermark is also an important factor in telemedicine applications. Therefore, watermarking methods using encryption techniques should be simple to save execution time of encryption and decryption [36]. The text watermark in the proposed method is encrypted using the equation

$$Encrypted\ text = \left(input\ text^{r}\right) - d \tag{4.1}$$

where r and d are constants. Here, r can have a value in the range 1.000 to 1.143 and d can be between 0.0 and 10.0. The first level of security lies in this encryption process [37].

The extracted encrypted text is decrypted at the receiving end using the relation

$$Decrypted\ text = \left(Encrypted\ text + d\right)^{\frac{1}{r}} \tag{4.2}$$

4.6   Experimental Results and Performance Analysis

In this section, the performance of the combined DWT-DCT-SVD image watermarking method is first discussed. Subsequently, the performance of the watermarking scheme using image and text watermark as multiple watermarking is analyzed followed by discussion on improvements achieved by using multiple watermarking.

4.6.1   Performance Evaluation of the Proposed Method Using Image Watermark

The gray–level images "Barbara Image" of size 512×512 and "Thorax" of size 256×256 are used as cover and watermark images respectively. These images are shown in Fig. 4.1a, b, respectively. The proposed hybrid watermarking method was implemented in MATLAB. The watermarked image is shown in Fig. 4.1c. The imperceptibility of the hidden watermark and the robustness of the watermark were evaluated by determining PSNR and NC values, respectively. The robustness of the proposed method against different known attacks was compared with the robustness offered by methods proposed by Singh and Tayal [22], Khan et al. [23] and Harish et al. [25]. In the experiments, the gain factor (α) is taken as 0.01 and 0.1 for evaluating PSNR and NC performance with no attack. The highest PSNR = 55.01 dB was

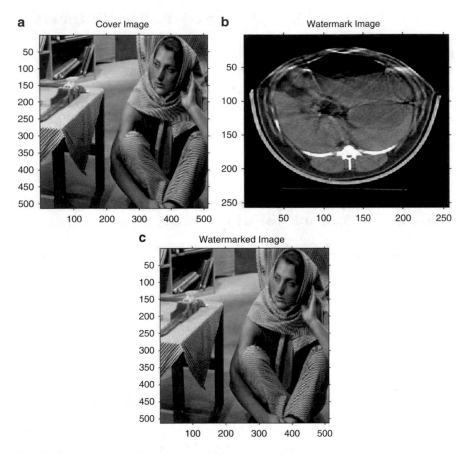

Fig. 4.1 Image (**a**) cover (**b**) watermark and (**c**) watermarked

obtained at the $\alpha = 0.01$ and the highest NC = 1 was obtained at $\alpha = 0.1$. However, with noise attacks the gain factor α was considered from 0.5 to 0.9. These values were taken for the comparison with other reported techniques.

The robustness performance (determined NC value) for the proposed method under different attacks is shown in Table 4.1. With reference to this table, NC values are shown for LL and HH sub-bands at different gain factors ($\alpha = 0.5, 0.7$ and 0.9). In addition, the table compares NC values for HH sub-band as obtained by the proposed method and as reported in [22] for the $\alpha = 0.5$. It may be observed that best results are obtained for LL sub-band against the Histogram equalization attack. The highest NC value = 0.9999 is obtained against this attack at $\alpha = 0.9$.

In Table 4.2, NC values are shown for Salt and pepper noise at noise densities from 0.01 to 0.08 and the obtained results demonstrate better performance for LL sub-band. It is observed that the NC value decreases as the noise density increases. The proposed method for HH sub-band provides better performance than that of the results reported by Singh and Tayal [22]. Even at high noise density of 0.08, the

Table 4.1 Effect of attacks on robustness (determined using NC values) at different wavelet decomposition levels

Attacks	NC values (proposed method using Haar Wavelet) LL sub-band α = 0.9	NC values (proposed method using Haar Wavelet) LL sub-BAND α = 0.7	NC values (proposed method using Haar Wavelet) LL sub-band α = 0.5	NC values (proposed method using Haar Wavelet) HH sub-band α = 0.5	NC values [22] (Singh and Tayal method using Haar Wavelet) HH sub-band α = 0.5
Sobel horizontal edge emphasizing filter	0.9996	0.9994	0.9994	0.9992	0.9992
Linear motion	0.9979	0.9985	0.9996	0.9927	0.9912
Disk (circular averaging filter)	0.9979	0.9989	0.9996	0.9887	0.9887
Average filter[3 3], Average filter[5 5], Average filter[7 7]	0.9979, 0.9909, 0.9896	0.9934, 0.9900, 0.9894	0.9926, 0.9898, 0.9893	0.9914, 0.9897, 0.9891	0.9909, 0.9896, 0.9891
Poisson noise	0.9981	0.9974	0.9973	0.9811	0.9754
Contrast adjustment	0.9915	0.9886	0.9812	0.9558	0.9338
Histogram equalization	0.9999	0.9998	0.9996	0.9994	0.9991

Table 4.2 Effect of Salt and pepper noise on robustness (determined using NC values) at different wavelet decomposition levels

Noise density	NC values (proposed method using Haar Wavelet) LL sub-band α = 0.9	NC values (proposed method using Haar Wavelet) LL sub-band α = 0.7	NC values (proposed method using Haar Wavelet) LL sub-band α = 0.5	NC values (proposed method using Haar Wavelet) HH sub-band α = 0.5	NC values [22] (Singh and Tayal method using Haar Wavelet) HH sub-band α = 0.5
0.01	0.9962	0.9961	0.9948	0.9636	0.9636
0.02	0.9917	0.9910	0.9855	0.9295	0.9289
0.03	0.9869	0.9823	0.9719	0.9043	0.8971
0.04	0.9799	0.9734	0.9565	0.8804	0.8685
0.05	0.9729	0.9635	0.9439	0.8612	0.8420
0.06	0.9641	0.9508	0.9226	0.8430	0.8209
0.07	0.9551	0.9389	0.9059	0.8271	0.7980
0.08	0.9468	0.9277	0.8892	0.8171	0.7809

performance of the proposed method with HH sub-band at α = 0.5 gives NC value of 0.8171 against 0.7809 as obtained by [22]. However, the proposed method performs better with LL sub-band as it has higher NC value (= 0.8892) at the same gain factor.

In Table 4.3, NC values are shown for Gaussian noise at noise variance from 0.01 to 0.08 and the obtained results demonstrate better performance with LL sub-band. However, the proposed method with HH sub-band provides better performance than the results reported by Singh and Tayal [22]. Even at the high noise variance of 0.08, the performance of the proposed method with HH sub-band at $\alpha = 0.5$ gives NC value of 0.8894 against 0.6142 as obtained by [22]. However, the proposed method obtained better value of NC (= 0.9282) with LL sub-band at the same gain factor. An increase in gain factor (α) to 0.9 increases NC to 0.9523 with LL sub-band.

In Table 4.4, NC values have been evaluated for Speckle noise at noise variance from 0.01 to 0.08. The result shows the better performance with LL band. However,

Table 4.3 Effect of Gaussian noise on robustness (determined using NC values) at different wavelet decomposition levels

Variance	NC values (proposed method using Haar Wavelet) LL sub-band $\alpha = 0.9$	NC values (proposed method using Haar Wavelet) LL sub-band $\alpha = 0.7$	NC values (proposed method using Haar Wavelet) LL sub-band $\alpha = 0.5$	NC values (proposed method using Haar Wavelet) HH sub-band $\alpha = 0.5$	NC values [22] (Singh and Tayal method using Haar Wavelet) HH sub-band $\alpha = 0.5$
0.01	0.9872	0.9841	0.9752	0.8939	0..8893
0.02	0.9841	0.9818	0.9727	0.8937	0.8116
0.03	0.9803	0.9770	0.9689	0.8930	0.7563
0.04	0.9760	0.9730	0.9617	0.8925	0.7139
0.05	0.9709	0.9661	0.9531	0.8923	0.6814
0.06	0.9649	0.9593	0.9452	0.8919	0.6565
0.07	0.9587	0.9513	0.9336	0.8914	0.6323
0.08	0.9523	0.9441	0.9282	0.8894	0.6142

Table 4.4 Effect of Speckle noise on robustness (determined using NC values) at different wavelet decomposition levels

Variance	NC values (proposed method using Haar Wavelet) LL sub-band $\alpha = 0.9$	NC values (proposed method using Haar Wavelet) LL sub-band $\alpha = 0.7$	NC values (proposed method using Haar Wavelet) LL sub-band $\alpha = 0.5$	NC values (proposed method using Haar Wavelet) HH sub-band $\alpha = 0.5$	NC values [22] (Singh and Tayal method using Haar Wavelet) HH sub-band $\alpha = 0.5$
0.01	0.9981	0.9948	0.9944	0.9662	0.9662
0.02	0.9906	0.9896	0.9848	0.9660	0.9659
0.03	0.9849	0.9818	0.9724	0.9116	0.9057
0.04	0.9786	0.9727	0.9570	0.8903	0.8808
0.05	0.9718	0.9626	0.9405	0.8725	0.8569
0.06	0.9631	0.9496	0.9262	0.8557	0.8370
0.07	0.9540	0.9409	0.9078	0.8441	0.8191
0.08	0.9458	0.9275	0.8918	0.8323	0.8013

the proposed method with HH sub-band provides better performance than the results reported by Singh and Tayal [22]. Even at the high noise variance of 0.08, the performance of the proposed method with HH sub-band at gain factor $\alpha = 0.5$ gives NC value of 0.8323 against 0.8013 as obtained by [22]. However, the proposed method obtained better value of NC (= 0.8918) with LL sub-band at the same gain factor ($\alpha = 0.5$) and an increase in gain factor to 0.9 increases NC to 0.9458. Figure 4.2 shows NC performance of the proposed method against three different attcks (Salt & pepper, Gaussian and Speckle noise) at gain factor (α) = 0.9. Figure 4.3 shows the comparison of NC performance of the proposed method with the method reported by Singh and Tayal [22] at gain factor (α) = 0.5.

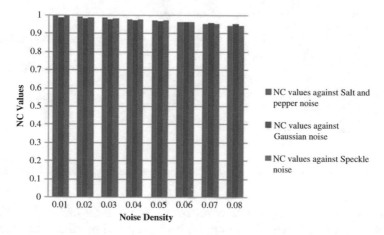

Fig. 4.2 NC performance of the proposed method against known attacks at gain factor (α) = 0.9

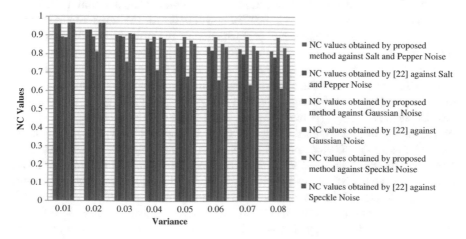

Fig. 4.3 Comparision of NC values with other reported method at gain factor (α) = 0.5

Table 4.5 Comparison of robustness (determined using NC values) performance with other reported methods

Attack	NC values (proposed method)	Max NC values (Khan et al. [23])	NC values (Harish et al. [25])
Gaussion noise	0.9872	0.9762	0.9690
Histogram equalization	0.9999	0.9979	0.9180
Salt and pepper noise	0.9962	0.9894	0.8940
Poisson noise	0.9981	0.9981	0.9390
Speckle noise	0.9981	0.9981	0.9890

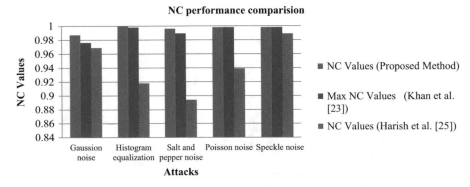

Fig. 4.4 Comparision of NC values with other reported methods [23, 25] against known attacks

Table 4.5 shows the comparison of robustness performance (determined NC values) of the proposed method with the methods proposed by Khan et al. [23] and Harish et al. [25]. It is observed that the maximum NC value obtained is highest for the proposed method. The maximum NC value with the proposed method is obtained as 0.9999 for the Histogram equalization attack. However, the maximum NC value has been obtained by [23, 25] are 0.9979 and 0.9180 for the same attack respectively. Figure 4.4 reveal better NC performance of the proposed method as compared to other methods [23, 25] in different wavelet decomposition level. The performance (determined NC values) of the proposed method is also tested by using the benchmark software 'Checkmark' [38, 39]. Table 4.6 shows the maximum NC values is obtained by the proposed method under twenty-four different 'Checkmark' attacks such as Collage, Trimmed Mean, Hard and Soft Thresholding, etc. at best performing gain factor with the value of 0.09. It may be observed from this table that the maximum NC value of 0.9774 has been obtained against projective attack. However, the minimum NC value is 0.6189 against rows and columns removal attack. Here, all the NC values are acceptable except the values obtained by the rows and columns removal, trimmed mean and mid-point attack as these are less than 0.7. Figure 4.5 shows the performance of the proposed method against different 'Checkmark' attacks. In general, it is observed that larger the gain factor, stronger is the robustness and smaller the gain factor, better is the image quality.

Table 4.6   Effect of 'Checkmark' attacks on robustness (determined using NC values) at gain factor (α) = 0.09

'Checkmark' attacks	Maximum NC values for image watermark
Collage	0.9003
Template remove	0.823
Rows and columns removal	0.6189
Denoising followed by perceptual remodulation (DPR)	0.7102
DPR_corr attack	0.7266
Scale	0.8753
Trimmed mean	0.643
Cropping	0.9829
Gaussian	0.8653
Hard thresholding	0.7777
Soft thresholding	0.7243
JPEG compression	0.7503
Wavelet compression	0.7146
Medium filter	0.8663
Mid point	0.689
Projective	0.9774
Linear	0.8816
Ratio	0.7912
Rotation scale	0.8224
Rotation	0.7547
Shearing	0.8787
Warp	0.8247
Wiener	0.7936
Sampledownup	0.756

4.6.2   Performance Evaluation of the Proposed Method Using Multiple Watermarks

The performance of the proposed watermarking method has also been evaluated for embedding multiple watermarks (image and text) in the cover image. The proposed method uses medical image as the image watermark, and the personal and medical record of the patient as the text watermark for identity authentication purpose. Figure 4.6a, b show multiple watermark embedding and extraction processes. For testing the robustness and quality of the watermarked image MATLAB is used. In the proposed method cover image of size 512×512, the image watermark of size 256×256 and the text watermark of size 50 characters are used for testing. The robustness of the image and text watermarks is evaluated by determining NC and BER, respectively. The quality of watermarked image is evaluated by PSNR.

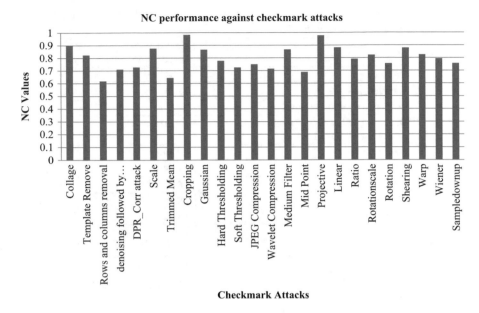

NC performance against checkmark attacks

Fig. 4.5 Robustness performance of the proposed method against 'Checkmark' attacks

It is quite apparent that size of the watermark affects quality of the watermarked image. The size of the watermark is sum total of bits occupied by all watermarks in the case of multiple watermarking. However, degradation in quality of the watermarked image will not be observable if the size of watermark (total size in case of multiple watermarking) is small. Figure 4.7a shows the CT Scan cover image and Fig. 4.7b–d show watermarked images at different gain factors 0.05, 0.5 and 1.0 respectively. Figure 4.8a shows the original image watermark (Thorax image). The image watermark embedding method is based on DWT, DCT and SVD. The text watermark is the patient data as shown in Fig. 4.8b.

In order to enhance security of the text watermark encryption is applied to the ASCII representation of the text watermark before embedding. The image and text watermarks are embedded using the methods described in Sect. 4.2. The performance of the proposed method is determined by varying the gain factor, size of the text watermark, and cover images. It is found that larger gain factor results in stronger robustness of the extracted watermark whereas smaller gain factor provides better PSNR values between original and watermarked medical images. Experimental results illustrate that the proposed method is able to withstand a variety of signal processing attacks. The following observations are apparent:

(i) *Capacity of embedding multiple watermark*: The methods proposed in [16–18, 22–25, 40, 41] embed only single watermark. However, in the proposed method multiple watermarks (text and image) are embedded simultaneously, which provides extra level of security with acceptable performance in terms of robustness

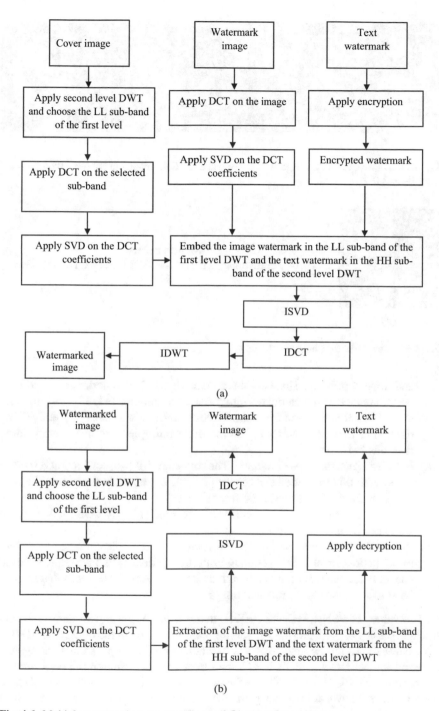

Fig. 4.6 Multiple watermarks (**a**) embedding and (**b**) extraction process

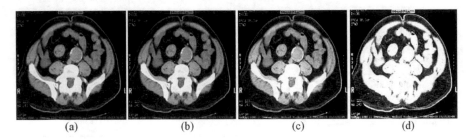

(a)   (b)   (c)   (d)

Fig. 4.7 (**a**) Cover CT Scan image and Watermarked CT Scan images at (**b**) $\alpha = 0.05$ (**c**) $\alpha = 0.5$ and (**d**) $\alpha = 1.0$

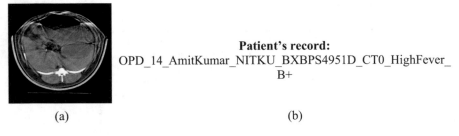

Patient's record:
OPD_14_AmitKumar_NITKU_BXBPS4951D_CT0_HighFever_
B+

(a)   (b)

Fig. 4.8 Watermarks (**a**) Image and (**b**) Text

and imperceptibility. There are three methods for dual watermark embedding, we can embed two watermarks either one after another [42, 43] or simultaneously [44]. It is reported that simultaneous multiple watermarking embedding method has fewer constraints than the other multiple watermarks embedding methods [44].

(ii) *Improved robustness performance*: The robustness of proposed method is compared with other reported techniques [22, 24, 28] and it is found that the proposed method offers superior performance.

(iii) *Enhance the security*: The security of the medical text watermark may be enhanced by using encryption.

(iv) *Reduced storage and bandwidth requirements*: The medical image files / electronic patient record (EPR) contain important patient data. Further, in order to conserve the transmission bandwidth or storage space the patient's details may be embedded inside the medical image.

The values of PSNR, NC and BER as determined by the experiments are illustrated in Tables 4.7, 4.8 and 4.9 for varying gain factor (α) in the range of 0.01–0.5. Figure 4.9 shows the NC and BER value obtained by the proposed method against different known attacks. In Table 4.7, the effect of encryption on the performance (determined PSNR, NC and BER) of the proposed method against different sizes of watermark is shown at different gain factors. With encryption, maximum PSNR value obtained by the proposed method is 35.84 dB. The maximum NC value obtained with encryption is 0.9992 at gain factor (α) = 0.1. The BER = '0' is obtained with encryption at all chosen gain factors. However, the BER = 0.08 is obtained

Table 4.7 Effect of encryption on PSNR, NC and BER at different gain factors

Gain factor (α)	Without encryption						With encryption					
	Text watermark size = 50 characters			Text watermark size = 30 characters			Text watermark size = 50 characters			Text watermark size = 30 characters		
	PSNR (dB)	NC values	BER (%)	PSNR (dB)	NC values	BER (%)	PSNR (dB)	NC values	BER (%)	PSNR (dB)	NC values	BER (%)
0.01	35.84	0.9808	0.08	36.19	0.9808	0.02	35.84	0.9802	0	36.19	0.9801	0
0.05	34.64	0.9986	0.08	34.9	0.9989	0.02	34.64	0.9985	0	34.9	0.9988	0
0.10	32.19	0.9992	0.08	32.34	0.9993	0	32.19	0.9992	0	32.34	0.9993	0

Table 4.8 NC and BER performance of the proposed method against different attacks at gain factor (α) = 0.05

Attacks	Proposed method With encryption	
	Image watermark (NC value)	Text watermark (BER value in %)
JPEG compression (QF = 10)	0.9905	0.96
JPEG compression (QF = 50)	0.9785	0.62
JPEG compression (QF = 90)	0.9982	0
Median filtering [1 1] and [2 2]	0.9985, 0.9752	0, 0.93
Scaling factor 2	0.7375	0.44
Scaling factor 1.5	0.8086	0.26
Scaling factor 1.1	0.8964	0
Gaussian LPF (standard deviation = 0.6 and 0.4)	0.9343, 0.9913	0.36, 0
Gaussian noise (mean = 0,Var = 0.01)	0.7267	0.5
Gaussian noise (mean = 0,Var = 0.001)	0.9365	0
Salt & pepper noise (density = 0.01)	0.7552	0.14
Salt & pepper noise (density = 0.05)	0.6069	0.48
Salt & pepper noise (density = 0.001)	0.9843	0
Histogram equalization	0.569	0.14

Table 4.9 PSNR and NC performance using different cover images at gain factor (α) = 0.05

Image type	Using encryption		
	PSNR (dB)	NC value	BER
Brain	35.61	0.9743	0.5
CT Scan	34.64	0.9985	0
Ultrasound	37.62	0.9983	0.6
MRI	35.78	0.9960	0.64
Lena	37.23	0.9998	0.02
Barbara	28.35	0.9997	0

without encryption at all chosen gain factors. Table 4.8 shows the performance (determined NC and BER values) of the proposed watermarking method against different attacks. With encryption, the highest BER value of 0.96 has been obtained against JPEG Compression attack with quality factor (QF) = 10. The performance of the proposed method was also determined with six different cover images i.e. Brain, CT Scan, Ultrasound, MRI, Lena and Barbara.

Figure 4.10 shows the PSNR, NC and BER value obtained by the proposed method for different cover images. Table 4.9 shows the PSNR, NC and BER values obtained by the proposed method with encryption for these different cover images at gain factor (α) = 0.05. The highest PSNR = 37.62 dB was obtained with Ultrasound image. Here, the NC and BER values obtained were 0.9983 and 0.6 respectively. However, the maximum NC and BER were obtained with Lena and MRI image,

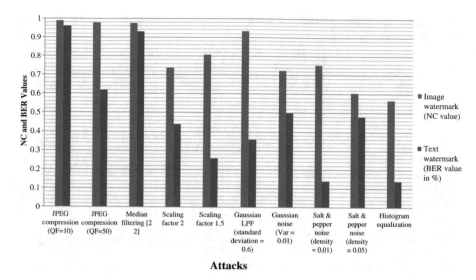

Fig. 4.9 NC and BER performance of the proposed method against different attacks

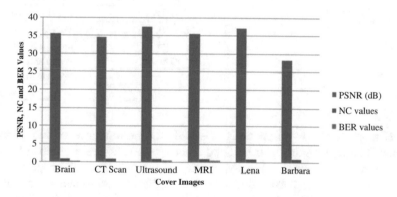

Fig. 4.10 PSNR, NC and BER performance of the proposed method using different cover images

respectively. In Table 4.10 the robustness performance (determined NC values) of the proposed method against eight different attacks is compared with robustness offered by other methods as reported in [22, 24, 28]. It is observed that the proposed method offers higher robustness against all these attacks as compared to these methods. The NC values with the proposed method are obtained as 0.9994, 0.9752 and 0.6565 against JPEG, Median Filtering, and Gaussian noise (Var-0.5) attacks, respectively. The NC values obtained with the proposed method are 0.9956, 0.9754, 0.9952, 0.8856 and 0.9208 against Gaussian low pass filter (LPF), Gaussian noise (Var-0.01), Salt & pepper Noise (Density = 0.01), Salt & pepper noise (Density = 0.08)

Table 4.10 Performance comparison of robustness (determined using NC values) performance under different attacks

Attacks	Singh and Tayal [22]	Srivastav et al. [24]	Rosiyadi et al. [28]	Proposed method
JPEG compression (QF = 50)	Not reported	Not reported	−0.1863	0.9994
Median filtering [2 2]	Not reported	0.6019	0.4585	0.9752
Gaussian LPF	0.9956	Not reported	Not reported	0.9956
Gaussian noise (mean = 0,Var = 0.5)	Not reported	Not reported	0.5012	0.6565
Gaussian noise (mean = 0,Var = 0.01)	0.8893	0.632	Not reported	0.9754
Salt & pepper noise (density = 0.08)	0.7809	Not reported	Not reported	0.8856
Histogram equalization	0.9941	0.9123	Not reported	0.9208
Salt & pepper noise (density = 0.01)	0.9636	Not reported	Not reported	0.9952

Table 4.11 Subjective measure of the watermarked image quality at different gain factors

Gain factor (α)	Quality of the watermarked image
0.001	Excellent quality
0.01	Very good quality
0.05	Good quality
0.5	Average quality
1	Poor quality
5	Very poor quality

and Histogram attacks respectively. Overall, the performance of the proposed method is better than the other reported technique [22, 24, 28] in terms of robustness, capacity and security. Finally, quality of the watermarked image has been measured by the subjective method [45]. One medical specialist and two colleagues were involved to check and vote for the quality of the watermarked data. Table 4.11 reports their combined suggestion. It may be observed that the reported visual quality of the watermarked images is acceptable for diagnosis at all chosen gain factors except the gain factor (α) = 1.0 and 5.0, which indicate the poor quality. It may be concluded from the subjective measure test that smaller gain factor provides acceptable quality of the watermarked image for diagnosis.

From the above discussion, we have observed that the robustness of the watermark was experimentally determined by calculating NC values at different gain factors ('α') by applying known attacks as shown in Tables 4.1, 4.2, 4.3, 4.4 and 4.5 at different wavelet decomposition levels. Referring these tables, it is evident that the proposed algorithm offers up to 11.43% enhancement in NC value (i.e. robustness) as compared to the other reported techniques. Further, the NC values under different attacks using benchmark software 'Checkmark' are shown in Table 4.6 from which it is found that suggested technique is robust against the 'Checkmark' attacks except for NC values for rows and columns removal, trimmed mean and midpoint attacks where NC values are less than 0.7. The performance of suggested technique in respect of robustness and imperceptibility using multiple watermarking (image and text) has been evaluated in Sect. 4.4.2 for its utility in identity authentication. The suggested method of watermarking also offers capability of embedding multiple watermarks. Further, the proposed technique enhances security of the text watermark by encrypting it before embedding. A simple encryption method is used to keep small overhead of encryption/decryption of text watermark in terms of execution time. As shown in Table 4.10, the proposed method offers up to six times enhancement in robustness over other reported techniques.

4.6.3   Performance Evaluation of the Improved Hybrid Algorithm Using Multiple Watermarks

In order to improving the robustness and embedding capacity performance of the previous watermarking method (as discussed in Sect. 4.6.2) using multiple watermarks, the watermark image is transformed by DWT, DCT and SVD instead of DCT and DWT. The S vector of watermark information is embedded in the S component of the cover image. The watermarked image is generated by inverse SVD on modified S vector and original U, V vectors followed by inverse DCT and inverse DWT. The method has been extensively tested and analyzed against known attacks and is found to be giving superior performance for robustness, capacity and reduced storage and bandwidth requirements compared to reported techniques suggested by other authors. For the improved hybrid algorithm, the watermark embedding and extraction algorithm are presented in Fig. 4.11a, b respectively. The performance of the improved hybrid watermarking method by applying encryption on patient data before embedding into the cover has been investigated. In the improved method, cover image and the image watermark of size 512× 512 and the text watermark of size up to 185 characters are used for testing. In this method, the EPR as text watermarks are broadly classified as follows [46]:

i. Patient image/health centre logo watermark is embedded in the first level of the DWT image for the purpose of data integrity control.
ii. Patient's medical records/identity/reference watermark contains the physician's identification code, keywords and patient's personal and examination data. The physician's identification code is for the purpose of origin authentication.
iii. The keywords such as diagnostic codes, the insertion of indices image, acquisition characteristics, which facilitates image retrieval by database querying mechanisms. The efficient indexing and archiving of digital medical data in hospital information systems eliminates the storage and transmission bandwidth requirements.

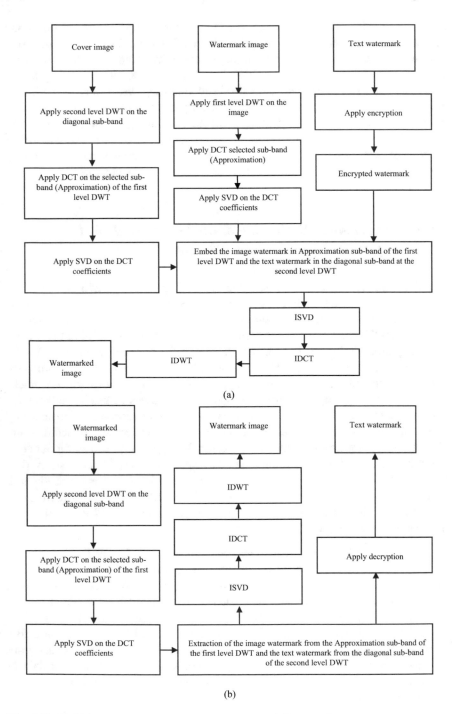

Fig. 4.11 Multiple watermarks (a) embedding process and (b) extraction process

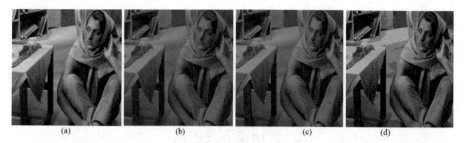

Fig. 4.12 (**a**) Cover image and (**b**) Watermarked Barbara images at gain factor = 0.05, (**c**) 0.1 and (**d**) 0.9

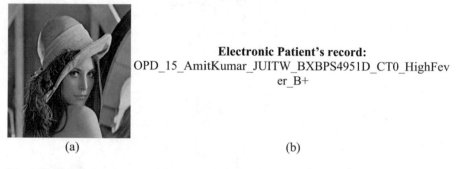

Electronic Patient's record:
OPD_15_AmitKumar_JUITW_BXBPS4951D_CT0_HighFev
er_B+

(a)   (b)

Fig. 4.13 Original (**a**) image and (**b**) text watermark of size 50 characters

It is quite apparent that size of the watermark affects quality of the watermarked image. The size of the watermark is sum total of bits occupied by all watermarks in the case of multiple watermarking. However, degradation in quality of the water-marked image will not be observable if the size of watermark (total size in case of multiple watermarking) is small. The image watermark (Lena image) embedding method is based on DWT, DCT and SVD. In order to enhance the security of the text watermark, encryption is applied to the ASCII representation of the text water-mark before embedding. Figure 4.12 shows the Barbara cover image and Fig. 4.12b–d show watermarked images at different gain factors 0.05, 0.1 and 0.9, respectively. Figure 4.13a shows the original image watermark (Lena image). The text water-mark is the patient data as shown in Fig. 4.13b. In the experiment, values of PSNR, NC and BER are illustrated in Tables 4.1, 4.2, 4.3 and 4.4 at varying gain factor (α) in the range of 0.01 to 0.1. In addition, the performance (PSNR, NC and BER) of the proposed method has been compared in Table 4.12 to Table 4.13. In Table 4.12, PSNR, NC and BER performance of the proposed hybrid method for different size of watermark has been evaluated without any noise attack. With the encryption, maximum PSNR value is 28.51 dB and BER = 0 against maximum size of water-mark at gain factor = 0.01. Here, the NC value is 0.9930. However, the maximum NC value is 1.0 at gain factor = 0.1. In addition, this table shows the PSNR, NC and

Table 4.12 Comparison under PSNR, NC and BER with other reported technique at different gain factor

Gain factor (α)	Using encryption [47]						Proposed method using encryption					
	50 characters			30 characters			50 characters			30 characters		
	PSNR (dB)	NC values	BER (%)	PSNR (dB)	NC values	BER (%)	PSNR (dB)	NC values	BER (%)	PSNR (dB)	NC values	BER (%)
0.01	35.84	0.9802	0	36.19	0.9801	0	28.51	0.993	0	29.65	0.9937	0
0.05	34.64	0.9985	0	34.9	0.9988	0	28.12	0.999	0	29.43	0.9995	0
0.1	32.19	0.9992	0	32.34	0.9993	0	27.87	1	0	27.03	0.9998	0

Table 4.13 Comparison under NC and BER with other reported technique against attacks

Attacks	Singh et al. [47] method using encryption		Proposed method using encryption	
	Image watermark	Text watermark	Image watermark	Text watermark
	(NC value)	(BER value in %)	(NC value)	(BER value in %)
JPEG compression (QF-10)	0.9905	0.96	0.9913	0.48
JPEG compression (QF-50)	0.9785	0.62	0.9708	0
JPEG compression (QF-90)	0.9982	0	0.9993	0
Median filtering [1 1] and [2 2]	0.9985 and 0.9752	0 and 0.93	0.9993 and 0.9479	0 and 0.94
Scaling factor 1.1	0.8964	0	0.7251	0
Gaussian LPF with standard deviation = 0.6 and 0.4	0.9343 and 0.9913	0.36 and 0	0.8635 and 0.9959	0
Gaussian noise with mean = 0,Var-0.01	0.7267	0.5	0.6297	0
Gaussian noise with mean = 0,Var-0.001	0.9365	0	0.9591	0
Salt & Pepper noise (density = 0.01)	0.7552	0.14	0.7881	0
Salt & Pepper noise (density = 0.05)	0.6069	0.48	0.5919	0
Salt & Pepper noise (density = 0.001)	0.9843	0	0.9938	0
Histogram equalization	0.569	0.14	0.8157	0
Unsharp contrast enhancement filter ALPHA = 0.1, 0.2 and 0.5	Not reported	Not reported	0.6201, 0.6244 and 0.6341	0
Motion Blur (len = 1 and theta = 0)	Not reported	Not reported	0.9993	0
Motion Blur (len = 2 and theta = 0)	Not reported	Not reported	0.8619	0
Motion Blur (len = 2.5 and theta = 0)	Not reported	Not reported	0.8289	0.9

BER performance comparison of the proposed method with other reported techniques [47].

At this point, the maximum NC value with proposed method has been obtained as 0.9930, 0.9990 and 1.0 at gain factor 0.01, 0.05 and 0.1 respectively with acceptable PSNR values. However, the maximum NC value obtained with Singh et al. [47] method is 0.9802, 0.9995 and 0.9992 at the same gain factors, respectively. The BER value is zero in all the cases. The maximum PSNR value have been obtained with Singh et al. [47] is 35.84 dB at gain = 0.01 using the image watermark of size 256×256. However, the maximum PSNR value has been obtained by the proposed method is 28.51 dB at the same gain using the image watermark of size 512×512. The degradation in the PSNR value will be high if the size of image watermark (512×512) and the text watermark (50 Characters = 350 bits) is small.

Table 4.14 Effect of cover image at gain = 0.05

Image type	Singh et al. [47] using encryption			Proposed method using encryption		
	PSNR (dB)	NC value	BER (%)	PSNR (dB)	NC Value	BER (%)
Brain	35.61	0.9743	0.5	31.11	0.9894	0.2
CT Scan	34.64	0.9985	0	30.27	0.9984	0.12
Ultrasound	37.62	0.9983	0.6	31.15	0.9986	0.6
MRI	35.78	0.996	0.64	30.27	0.9984	0.1
Lena	37.23	0.9998	0.02	31.06	0.9998	0.01
Barbara	28.35	0.9997	0	26.86	0.9994	0

Table 4.15 Effect of size of the text watermark at gain = 0.01

Size of text watermark	PSNR (dB)	NC values	BER (%)
75 characters	27.69	0.9938	0
155 characters	27.43	0.9932	0
185 characters	27.38	0.9931	0.4

Table 4.13 shows the NC and BER performance of the proposed hybrid watermarking method for different attacks at gain factor = 0.05. With encryption, the maximum NC value of 0.9993 has been obtained against median filtering and Motion Blur attacks. However, minimum NC value of 0.5919 has been obtained against Salt & Pepper Noise (density = 0.05). The maximum BER value of 0.94 has been obtained against Median Filtering attacks. In addition, Table 4.2 shows the performance comparison of the proposed method with other reported techniques [47]. In this table, the maximum NC value with proposed method has been obtained as 0.9993, 0.9993, 0.9959, 0.9591, 0.9938, 0.8157, 0.6341, 0.993 against JPEG (QF = 90), median filtering, Gaussian low pass filter (standard deviation = 0.4), Gaussian noise (Var-0.001), Salt & Pepper noise (density = 0.001), Histogram equalization, Unsharp contrast enhancement filter (ALPHA = 0.5) and motion blur (len = 1 and theta = 0) attacks respectively. However, the maximum NC value obtained with Singh et al. [47] method is 0.9982, 0.9985, 0.9913, 0.9365, 0.9843 and 0.569 against JPEG (QF = 90), Median Filtering, Gaussian low pass filter (standard deviation = 0.4), Gaussian Noise (Var-0.001), Salt & Pepper Noise (density = 0.001), Histogram equalization attacks respectively. The BER value with proposed method is always zero except for JPEG Compression (QF-10), Median Filtering (2 2) and Motion Blur (len = 2.5 and theta = 0). However, the BER value with Singh et al. [47] is always greater than 0.14 except for JPEG Compression (QF-90), Median Filtering (1 1), Scaling (Factor = 1.1), Gaussian LPF (standard deviation = 0.4), Gaussian Noise (Var-0.001) and Salt & Pepper Noise (density = 0.001).

Table 4.14 shows the effect of cover image as proposed method was tested for other types of cover images like Brain, CT Scan, ultrasound, MRI, Lena and Barbara images. In addition, Table 4.14 shows the PSNR, NC and BER performance comparison of the proposed method with other reported techniques [47]. In this table, the maximum NC value with proposed method has been obtained as 0.9998 for Lena image, where the BER = 0.01. However, the same NC value with Singh et al. [40]

Table 4.16 Performance comparison results under NC value

Attacks	Singh and Tayal [22]	Srivastav and Saxena [24]	Rosiyadi et al. [28]	Proposed method
JPEG compression (QF = 50)	Not reported	Not reported	-0.1863	0.9988
Median filtering [2 2]	Not reported	0.6019	0.4585	0.9379
Gaussian LPF	0.9956	Not reported	Not reported	0.9959
Gaussian noise with mean = 0,Var-0.5	Not Found	Not reported	0.5012	0.6569
Gaussian noise with mean = 0,Var-0.01	0.8893	0.632	Not reported	0.9604
Salt & Pepper noise with (density = 0.08)	0.7809	Not reported	Not reported	0.8859
Histogram	0.9941	0.9123	Not reported	0.931
Salt & Pepper noise with density = 0.01	0.9636	Not reported	Not reported	0.9961

method has been obtained for Lena image, where the BER = 0.02. This Table shows that all the NC values are better than the technique proposed in [47] for all the selected images. In addition, the BER performance is also better than the existing method [47] except for the CT Scan image. Table 4.15 shows the PSNR, NC and BER performance of the proposed method for the different size of text watermark at gain = 0.01. This Table shows that the proposed method can embed up to 185 characters with acceptable PSNR value. However, the method can recovered up to 184 characters without any error. The proposed method can embed up to 184 characters. However, only 50 characters can be embedded by the method in [47]. Table 4.16 shows the performance comparison of the proposed method with other reported techniques [22, 24, 28]. In this table, the NC value with proposed method has been obtained as 0.9988, 0.9379 and 0.6569 against JPEG, Median Filtering, and Gaussian Noise (Var-0.5) attacks respectively. However, the NC value obtained with Rosiyadi et al. [28] method is - 0.1863, 0.4585 and 0.5012 against the same attacks respectively. The NC value with Singh and Tayal method [22] has been obtained as 0.9956, 0.8893, 0.7809 and 0.9636 against Gaussian LPF, Gaussian Noise (Var-0.01), Salt & Pepper Noise (density = 0.08) and Histogram attacks respectively. However, the NC value obtained with proposed method is 0.9959, 0.9604, 0.8859 and 0.931 against the same attacks respectively. The NC value with Srivastav and Saxena [24] has been obtained as 0.6019, 0.632 and 0.9123 against Median Filtering, Gaussian Noise (Var-0.01) and Histogram attacks respectively. However, the NC value obtained with proposed method is 0.9379, 0.9604 and 0.931 against the same attacks respectively.

From the above extensive discussions, it is found that larger gain factor results in stronger robustness of the extracted watermark whereas smaller gain factor provides better PSNR values between original and watermarked medical images. The performance of the proposed method is more robust than the other reported technique [47] in terms of robustness, capacity and BER. However, the reported technique [47] is much better than the other existing techniques [22, 24, 28]. Finally, the proposed method offer better performance (NC and BER values) compared to other reported techniques [22, 24, 28, 47].

4.7 Summary

In this chapter, the objective of this work is to develop watermarking methods that offer a good trade-off between major parameters i.e. imperceptibility, robustness, security, and capacity because it is difficult to have a single watermarking technique that can provide satisfactory performance of all parameters simultaneously. This chapter presented some improved methods of offering higher robustness using hybrid watermarking is proposed. The proposed methods simultaneously use of DWT, DCT and SVD to enhance watermark robustness. The imperceptibility of hidden watermark and its robustness were evaluated by determining PSNR and NC values, respectively. The performance of the proposed method is examined for known attacks including 'Checkmark' attacks. In addition, the performance of the proposed method has also been evaluated for multiple watermarking (image and text). The main features of discussed works in the chapter are identified as follows:

- The proposed watermarking technique using fusion of DWT, DCT, and SVD achieves better performance in terms of imperceptibility, robustness and capacity as compared to DWT, DCT and SVD applied individually or the combination of DWT-SVD/DCT-SVD.
- For identity authentication purposes, multiple watermarks have been embedded instead of single watermark into the same medical image/multimedia objects simultaneously, which offer superior performance in tele-medicine and tele-diagnosis applications. In the proposed method, two watermarks are embedded simultaneously.
- The proposed method offers significant enhancement in robustness, capacity and security at the acceptable visual quality over the existing techniques.
- Security of the text watermark is enhanced by using encryption. Encryption of EPR data before watermarking may have become unavoidable in recent tele-medicine application but the delay encountered during embedding and extraction will be an important factor. In the proposed method simple encryption algorithm is used to save execution time during embedding and extraction processes.
- Further, multiple watermarking in medical applications reduces the bandwidth and storage requirements, and acting as keywords for efficient achieving and fast data retrieval from querying mechanisms take place.

Overall, the proposed method is better than the other reported methods in terms of robustness, capacity and security. However, the performance of the proposed watermarking method highly depends on the size of the watermarks, gain factor and the noise variation. The proposed watermarking technique provides a valuable solution to the problem of patient identity theft and health data management issues in telemedicine applications.

References

1. L. Der-Chyuan, S. Chia-Hung, Robust image watermarking based on hybrid transformation, in Proceedings of IEEE International Carnahan Conference on Security Technology, Taiwan, pp. 394–399, 2003
2. M. Ouhsain, E.E. Abdallah, A. Ben Hamza, An image watermarking scheme based on wavelet and multiple-parameter fractional fourier transform, in Proceedings of IEEE International Conference on Signal Processing and Communications, Dubai, United Arab Emirates, pp. 1375–1378, 2007
3. M. Jiansheng, L. Sukang, T. Xiaomei, A digital watermarking algorithm based On DCT and DWT, in Proceedings of International Symposium on Web Information Systems and Applications, Nanchang, P. R. China, pp. 104–107, 2009
4. A.S. Hadi, B.M. Mushgil, H.M. Fadhil, Watermarking based Fresnel transform, wavelet transform, and chaotic sequence. J. Appl. Sci. Res. 5(10), 1463–1468 (2009)
5. C. Cao, R. Wang, M. Huang, R. Chen, A new watermarking method based on DWT and Fresnel diffraction transforms, in Proceedings of IEEE International Conference on Information Theory and Information Security, Beijing, pp. 433–430, 2010
6. C.-C. Lai, C.-C. Tsai, Digital image watermarking using discrete wavelet transform and singular value decomposition. IEEE Trans. Instrum. Meas. 59(11), 3060–3063 (2010)
7. A.A. Nakhaie, S.B. Shokouhi, No reference medical image quality measurement based on spread spectrum and discrete wavelet transform using ROI processing, in Proceedings of 24th Canadian Conference on Electrical and Computer Engineering, pp. 121–125, 2011
8. V.K. Ahire, V. Kshirsagar, Robust watermarking scheme based on discrete wavelet transform (DWT) and discrete cosine transform (DCT) for copyright protection of digital images. IJCSNS Int.J. Comput. Sci. Network Security 11(8), 208–213 (2011)
9. A. Umaamaheshvari, K. Thanushkodi, High performance and effective watermarking scheme for medical images. Eur. J. Sci. Res. 67(2), 283–293 (2012)
10. M. Soliman, A.E. Hassanien, N.I. Ghali, H.M. Onsi, An adaptive watermarking approach for medical imaging using swarm intelligent. Int. J. Smart Home 6(1), 37–50 (2012)
11. M.A. Hajjaji, E.-B. Bourennane, A.B. Abdelali, A. Mtibaa, Combining Haar Wavelet and Karhunen Loeve transforms for medical images watermarking. Biomed. Res. Int. 2014, 1–15 (2014)
12. A. Kannammal, S. Subha Rani, Two level security for medical images using watermarking/encryption algorithms. Int. J. Imaging Syst. Technol. 24(1), 111–120 (2014)
13. A. Al-Haj, A. Amer, Secured telemedicine using region-based watermarking with tamper localization. J. Digit. Imaging 27(6), 737–750 (2014)
14. S. Priya, B. Santhi, P. Swaminathan, Study on medical image watermarking techniques. J. Appl. Sci. 14(14), 1638–1642 (2014)
15. L. Gao, T. Gao, G. Sheng, S. Zhang, Robust medical image watermarking scheme with rotation correction, in Intelligent Data Analysis and Its Applications, Vol. 2, Advances in Intelligent Systems and Computing, ed. by J.-S. Pan et al. (Eds), vol. 298, (2014), pp. 283–292
16. N.H. Divecha, N.N. Jani, Image watermarking algorithm using DCT, DWT and SVD. Proc. Natl. Conf. Innov. Paradigms Eng. Technol. 10, 13–16 (2012)
17. K.A. Navas, A.M. Cheriyan, M. Lekshmi, S. Archana Tampy, M. Sasikumar, DWT–DCT–SVD based watermarking, in Proceedings of the 3rd International Conference on Communication Systems Software and Middleware and Workshop, Bangalore, pp. 271–274, 2008
18. B. Wang, J. Ding, Q. Wen, X. Liao, C. Liu, An image watermarking algorithm based on DWT DCT and SVD, in IEEE International Conference on Network Infrastructure and Digital Content, Beijing, pp. 1034–1038, 2009
19. V. Kelkar, H. Shaikh, M.I. Khan, Analysis of robustness of hybrid digital image watermarking technique under various attacks. Int. J. Comput. Sci. Mobile Comput. 2(3), 137–143 (2013)
20. S. Madhesiya, S. Ahmed, Advanced technique of digital watermarking based on SVD–DWT–DCT and Arnold transform. Int. J. Adv. Res. Comput. Eng. Technol. 2(5), 1918–1923 (2013)

21. F. Golshan, K. Mohammadi, A hybrid intelligent SVD based perceptual shaping of a digital image watermark in DCT and DWT domain. Imaging Sci. J. **61**(1), 35–46 (2013)
22. A. Singh, A. Tayal, Choice of Wavelet from Wavelet Families for DWT–DCT–SVD Image Watermarking. Int. J. Comput. Appl. **48**(17), 9–14 (2012)
23. M.I. Khan, M.M. Rahman, M.I.H. Sarker, Digital watermarking for image authentication based on combined DCT, DWT, and SVD transformation. Int. J. Comput. Sci. **10**(5), 223–230 (2013)
24. A. Srivastava, P. Saxena, DWT-DCT-SVD based semi blind image watermarking using middle frequency band. IOSR J. Comput. Eng. **12**(2), 63–66 (2013)
25. N.J. Harish, B.B.S. Kumar, A. Kusagur, Hybrid robust watermarking techniques based on DWT, DCT, and SVD. Int. J. Adv. Electr. Electr. Eng. **2**(5), 137–143 (2013)
26. A.K. Singh, M. Dave, A. Mohan, *A Hybrid Algorithm for Image Watermarking Against Signal Processing Attack*, ed. by S. Ramanna, et al., in Proceedings of 7th Multi-Disciplinary International Workshop in Artificial Intelligence, Krabi-Thailand, Lecture Notes in Computer Science (LNCS), vol. 8271, pp. 235–246, 2013
27. D. Rosiyadi, S.-J. Horng, P. Fan, X. Wang, Copyright protection for e-government document images. IEEE Multimedia **19**(3), 62–73 (2012)
28. D. Rosiyadi, S.-J. Horng, N. Suryana, N. Masthurah, A comparison between the hybrid using genetic algorithm and the pure hybrid watermarking scheme. Int. J. Comput. Theory Eng. **4**(3), 329–331 (2012)
29. H. Shi-Jinn, D. Rosiyadi, T. Li, T. Takao, K.M.K. GuoM, A blind image copyright protection scheme for e-government. J. Vis. Commun. Image Represent. **24**(7), 1099–1105 (2013)
30. H. Shi-Jinn, D. Rosiyadi, P. Fan, X. Wang, M.K. Khan, An adaptive watermarking scheme for e-government document images. Multimed Tools Appl. **72**(3), 3085–3103 (2014)
31. M. Ali, C. WookAhn, P. Siarry, Differential evolution algorithm for the selection of optimal scaling factors in image watermarking. Special issue on advances in evolutionary optimization based image processing. Eng. Appl. Artif. Intell. **31**, 15–26 (2014)
32. A.K. Singh, M. Dave, A. Mohan, Robust and secure multiple watermarking in wavelet domain. A special issue on advanced signal processing technologies and systems for healthcare applications (ASPTSHA). J. Med. Imaging Health Inf. **5**(2), 406–414 (2015)
33. A. Zear, A.K. Singh, P. Kumar, A proposed secure multiple watermarking technique based on DWT, DCT and SVD for application in medicine. Multimedia Tools Appl. (2016). doi:10.1007/s11042-016-3862-8
34. A. Sharma, A.K. Singh, S.P. Ghrera, Robust and secure multiple watermarking technique for medical images. Wirel. Pers. Commun. **92**(4), 1611–1624 (2017)
35. N. Terzjia, M. Repges, K. Luck, W. Geisselhardt, Digital image watermarking using discrete wavelet transform: performance comparison of error correction codes, in Proceedings of IASTED, 2002
36. Y. Zaz, L. El Fadil, Protecting EPR data using cryptography and digital watermarking, in Proceeding of International Conference on Models of Information and Communication Systems, Rabat, 2010
37. K.A. Navas, S. Nithya, R. Rakhi, M. Sasikumar, Lossless watermarking in JPEG2000 for EPR Data Hiding, in Proceeding of IEEEEIT, Chicago, USA, pp. 697–702, 2007
38. http://watermarking.unige.ch/Checkmark/
39. S. Pereira, S. Voloshynovskiy, M. Madueño, S. Marchand-Maillet, T Pun, Second generation benchmarking and application oriented evaluation, in Proceeding of Information Hiding Workshop III, Pittsburgh, PA, USA, pp. 340–353, 2001
40. D. Kalman, A singularly valuable decomposition: the SVD of a matrix, The American University, February 13, 2002
41. B.L. Gunjal, R.R. Manthalkar, An overview of transform domain robust digital image watermarking algorithms. J. Emerg. Trends Comput. Inf. Sci. **2**(1), 13–16 (2011)
42. K. Wu, W. Yan, J. Du, A robust dual digital-image watermarking technique, in Proceeding of International conference on Computational Intelligence and Security Workshop, pp. 668–671, 2007

43. C. Chemak, M.S. Bouhlel, J.C. Lapayre, A new scheme of robust image watermarking: the double watermarking algorithm, in Proceeding of 2007 Summer Computer Simulation Conference, San Diego, California, USA, pp. 1201–1208, 2007
44. H. Shen, B. Chen, From single watermark to dual watermark: a new approach for image watermarking. Comput. Electr. Eng. 38(5), 1310–1324 (2012)
45. A.K. Singh, B. Kumar, S.K. Singh, S.P. Ghrera, A. Mohan, Multiple watermarking technique for securing online social network contents using Back Propagation Neural Network. Futur. Gener. Comput. Syst. (2016). doi:10.1016/j.future.2016.11.023
46. A.K. Singh, M. Dave, A. Mohan, Multilevel encrypted text watermarking on medical images using spread-spectrum in DWT domain. Wireless Personal Commun.: Int. J. 83(3), 2133–2150 (2015)
47. A.K. Singh, M. Dave, A. Mohan, Hybrid technique for robust and imperceptible multiple watermarking using medical images. J Multimedia Tools Appl. 75(14), 8381–8401 (2015)

Chapter 5
Robust and Secure Multiple Watermarking for Medical Images

Amit Kumar Singh, Basant Kumar, Ghanshyam Singh, and Anand Mohan

5.1 Introduction

Recently, tele-medicine, tele-ophthalmology, tele-diagnosis, tele-consultancy, tele-cardiology, tele-radiology applications play an important role in the development of the medical field. However, to protect transmission, storage and sharing of electronic patient record (EPR) data via unsecure channel are the most important issues for these applications [1]. These watermarks are difficult to remove by unauthorized person and are robust against known or accidental attacks [2]. The digital imaging and communications in medicine (DICOM) is a basic criterion to communicate EPR data. A header is attached with the DICOM medical image files which contain important information about the patient. However, this header may be lost, attacked or disordered and further the header needs additional bandwidth. Due to these reasons, the watermarking techniques provide alternative solution to the

A.K. Singh (✉)
Department of Computer Science & Engineering, Jaypee University
of Information Technology, Waknaghat, Solan, India
e-mail: amit_245singh@yahoo.com

B. Kumar
Department of Electronics and Communication Engineering,
Motilal Nehru National Institute of Technology, Allahabad, India
e-mail: singhbasant@yahoo.com

G. Singh
Department of Electronics and Communication Engineering, Jaypee University
of Information Technology, Waknaghat, Solan, India
e-mail: drghanshyam.singh@yahoo.com

A. Mohan
Department of Electronics Engineering, Indian Institute of Technology (BHU),
Varanasi, India
e-mail: profanandmohan@gmail.com

© Springer International Publishing AG 2017   95
A.K. Singh et al. (eds.), *Medical Image Watermarking*, Multimedia Systems
and Applications, DOI 10.1007/978-3-319-57699-2_5

transmission of medical images/patient data. The main advantages of the medical image watermarking [1–4] are discussed detail in chapter 1. The transmitted images are prone to corruption in the transmission medium due to noise. However, any distortion in the received images may lead to faulty watermark detection and inappropriate disease diagnosis. The use of ECCs not only addresses this problem but also enhances robustness of the watermark [2].

> *The rest of the chapter is organized as follows. The related and recent state-of-the-art techniques are provided in Sect. 5.2. Section 5.3 provides the main contribution of the proposed work. The proposed technique is detailed in Sect. 5.4. The experimental results and brief analysis of the work is reported in Sect. 5.5. Next, our summary of the chapter is presented in Sect. 5.6.*

5.2 Related Works

Brief overviews of recent and related watermarking methods are presented as follows. Dhanalakshmi and Thaiyalnayaki [5] proposed a dual watermarking method based on DWT-SVD and chaos encryption. In this method, the secondary watermark is embedded into primary watermark and the resultant watermarked image is encrypted using chaos based logistic map. Finally, the resultant watermarked image is embedded into the cover image and transmitted. The experimental results have demostrated that the method is robust against signal processing attacks. The method proposed in [6] embeds multiple watermarks in the cover image. In this embedding process, a digital signature is first embedded into logo image and then a signed logo is embedded into the cover image. Also, the pseudo random generator based on the mathematical constant π has been developed and used at different stages in the method. Singh et al. [7] proposed a watermarking method based on three different ECCs. Out of the three ECCs, the Reed-Solomon shows the best performance. Mahajan and Patil [8] proposed a dual watermarking method based on DWT and SVD. In the watermark embedding process, the secondary watermark is embedded into primary watermark first and then the combined watermark is embedded into the cover image. The robustness of this method has been tested by applying signal processing attacks. Lai and Tsai [9] proposed a hybrid image-watermarking scheme based on DWT and SVD. After the first level decomposition of the cover image by Haar wavelet, SVD is applied to selected sub-band only. Now, dividing the watermark image into two parts, singular values in high-low (HL) and low-high (LH) sub-band are modified with half of the watermark image and then SVD is applied over them. The watermark extraction is just reversing the embedding process. With SVD, small modification of singular values does not affect the visual recognition of the cover image, which improves the robustness and transparency of the method. However, the computational cost is high and the proposed method uses SVD transform technique that requires extra storage. Terzija et al. [10] proposed a method for improving the efficiency and robustness of the watermarks. Three different error correction codes, (15,7)-BCH, (7,4)-Hamming Code and (15-7)-Reed–Solomon code, are applied to the ASCII representation of the text watermark. For embedding process, the original image is first decomposed up to second level using the discrete wavelet transform and watermark is added to the selected DWT coefficients. Experimental results examined that Reed–Solomon code perform better in terms of reducing BER values and its excellent ability to correct errors. However, the method is unable to correct the error rates greater than 20%. Kumar et al. [11] have been proposed an algorithm for text watermark representing each character in binary format using ASCII codes. BCH code is used to enhance the bit error rate (BER) performance of the extracted watermark.

Giakoumaki et al. [12] presents a medical image watermarking technique using wavelet and BCH error correcting code. This method is embedding three water-marks in the form of signature, index, caption and reference at different decomposi-tion level and sub-bands of DWT cover image. For improving the robustness, BCH error correcting code is applied on the selected watermark before embedding into the cover medical image. Chang et al. [13] proposed an Integer wavelet transform (IWT) based multipurpose watermarking method in which authentication and robust watermarks are embedding into the selected wavelet coefficients. The IWT is easy to implement and has fast multiplication-free implementation. However, the IWT has poor energy compaction than common wavelet transforms. Kannammal et al. [14] have developed a medical image watermarking technique in which the water-mark is embedding into the selected sub-band of the natural cover image. Further, security of the watermarked is enhanced by using three different encryption tech-niques is applied on the watermarked image. The performance of these three encryp-tion techniques is compared in terms of time for encrypt and decrypt the massage. The experimental results established that the method is robust for different kind of attacks and the RC4 encryption technique perform better than the other two encryp-tion techniques.

5.3 Main Contribution of the Work

The method proposed in [9, 10] are embedding either text or image watermark. However, the multiple watermarking methods are more advantages for the medical applications. For the ownership identification purpose, the proposed hybrid method combined both reported techniques [9, 10] and embeds two watermarks (text and image) simultaneously [15–17] into the cover image. The objective of this chapter is to address the issue of channel noise distortions on watermark. The channel noise distortions may lead to faulty watermark and this could result into inappropriate disease diagnosis in telemedicine environment. This has been achieved using ECCs [18, 19] for encoding the watermark before embedding which is done using DWT and SVD. The effects of Hamming, BCH, Reed-Solomon and hybrid ECC consist-ing of BCH and repetition code on the robustness of text watermark and the cover image quality have been investigated in this chapter. The technique used to embed multiple watermarks is based on DWT and SVD. The proposed method is robust against known attacks without significantly degrading the image quality. Out of the four ECCs, it is found that the hybrid code shows the best performance. In addition, the performance of the proposed watermarking method by applying Reed-Solomon ECC on encrypted patient data before embedding the watermark has been investigated in section "Introduction". Further, the method is compared with other reported technique and has been found to be giving superior performance for robustness, security and capacity. Moreover, the robustness of the proposed method has been also tested using benchmark software 'Checkmark' and is found that this method is robust against the 'Checkmark' attacks.

5.4 Proposed Method

The watermark embedding and extraction process is shown in Fig. 5.1a, b respectively. In the embedding process, the cover image is decomposed at second level DWT. The image watermark is embedded into intermediate frequency sub-bands (HL and LH) of the first level DWT and the text watermark is embedded into higher coefficients sub-band (HH2) of the second level DWT. The hybrid proposed method has four parts, the image watermark embedding and extraction processes, and the text watermark embedding and extraction processes. The method proposed in [10] was modified to embed and extract text watermark. The details of four algorithms are given in separate subsections:

5.4.1 Embedding Algorithm for Image Watermark

The embedding algorithm for image watermark is formulated as follows: start:
STEP 1: Variable Declaration
Medical Image (MRI): Cover image
Leena: Watermark image
C_w: Read the cover image
W_w: Read the watermark image
α : Gain factor
DWT and SVD: Transform domain techniques
Wavelet filters: Haar
LL_c , HL_c , LH_c and HH_c : First level DWT coefficients for cover image
LL_{c1} , HL_{c1} , LH_{c1} and HH_{c1}: Second level DWT coefficients for cover image
S_{c1}: diagonal matrix for HL_c
S_{c2}: diagonal matrix for LH_c
U_{c1} and V_{c1}^T : orthonormal matrices for HL_c
U_{c2} and V_{c2}^T : orthonormal matrices for LH_c
α : Gain factor
W_w^k : modified value of S_{ck}

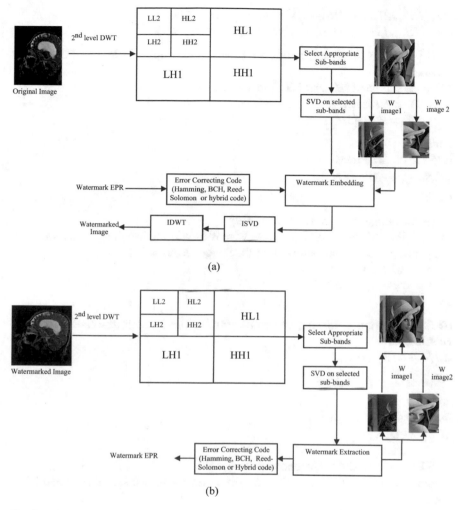

Fig. 5.1 The watermark (**a**) embedding and (**b**) extraction process

U_{cw}^{k} and V_{cw}^{kT} : orthonormal matrices for W_{w}^{k}

S_{cw}^{k} : diagonal matrix for W_{w}^{k}

W_{kmodi}: Modified DWT coefficient

W_{d}: Watermarked Image

STEP 2: Read the Images
M_w← MRI.bmp (Cover image of size 512 × 512)
L_w← Leena.bmp (Watermark image of size 256 × 256)

STEP 3: Perform DWT on Cover image
Apply second level DWT on cover image and first level DWT on Watermark image

$[LL_c, HL_c, LH_c$ and $HH_c] \leftarrow$ DWT (M_w, wavelet filter);
$[LL_{c1}, HL_{c1}, LH_{c1}$ and $HH_{c1}] \leftarrow$ DWT $(LL_c$, wavelet filter);

STEP 4: Choice of sub-bands in Cover and apply SVD on the selected sub-bands
//Choose sub-band HL_c and LH_c from cover image
if (SVD on HL_c)**then**
$$U_{c1}S_{c1}V_{c1}^T \leftarrow SVD(HL_c)$$
endif;
if (SVD on LH_c) **then**
$$U_{c2}S_{c2}V_{c2}^T \leftarrow SVD(LH_c)$$
endif;

STEP 5: Image Watermark Embedding
//Divide the watermark into two parts W = W1+W2, modify the singular values in HL_{c1} and LH_{c1} sub-bands with half of the image watermark
for $\alpha \leftarrow 0.01 : 0.1$
$S_{ck} + \alpha\, Wk = W_w^k$; k = 1, 2
end;

STEP 6: Compute the singular values for W_w^k and obtain the modified DWT coefficients
if $\left(SVD\, on\, W_w^k\right)$ **then**
$$[U_{cw}^k S_{cw}^k V_{cw}^{kT} \leftarrow SVD\left(W_w^k\right)$$
endif;
//modified DWT coefficient
$$W_{kmodi} \leftarrow U_{ck}S_{cw}^k V_{ck}^T$$

STEP 7: Obtain the Watermarked Image W_d
//Apply inverseDWT to LL_c , HL_c , LH_c and HH_c using two sets of modified DWT coefficients and
two sets of unmodified DWT coefficients.
$W_d \leftarrow$ inverse DWT(LL_c, HL_c, LH_c and HH_c, wavelet filter);
end:

5.4.2 Extraction Algorithm for Image Watermark

The extraction algorithm for image watermark is formulated as follows:
start:
STEP 1: Variable Declaration
α : gain factor
LL_c , HL_c , LH_c and HH_c: sub-bands for watermarked image
S_{cw1}: diagonal matrix for HL_c
S_{cw2}: diagonal matrix for LH_c
U_{cw1} and V_{cw1}^T : orthonormal matrices for HL_c

U_{cw2} and V_{cw2}^T : orthonormal matrices for LH_c
DW: modified singular value of selected sub-bands of cover image
Wk: extracted watermark
k : 1 and 2

STEP 2: Perform DWT on Watermarked image (possibly distorted)
$[LL_c, HL_c, LH_c$ and HH_c, wavelet filter$]\leftarrow$ DWT (W_d, wavelet filter);

STEP 3: Compute the singular values for HL_c and LH_c sub-bands
//Apply SVD to HL_c , LH_c sub-bands
if (SVD on HL_c)**then**
$U_{cw1}S_{cw1}V_{cw1}^T \leftarrow SVD(HL_c)$
endif;
if (SVD on LH_c) **then**
$U_{cw2}S_{cw2}V_{cw2}^T \leftarrow SVD(LH_c)$
endif;

STEP 4: Compute DW
//modify the singular value of cover image
$DW \leftarrow U_{cw}^k S_{cwk} V_{cw}^{kT}$; k = 1, 2

STEP 5: Extract the half of the watermark image from each sub-band and combined

$Wk = \dfrac{DW - S_{ck}}{\alpha}$; k = 1, 2

end:

5.4.3   Embedding Algorithm for Text Watermark

The embedding algorithm for text watermark is formulated as follows:

start:
STEP 1: Variable Declaration
Medical Image(MRI): cover image
C_w: read the cover image
W_w: read the text watermark
α : scale factor
DWT : discrete wavelet transforms
Wavelet filters: Haar
LL_c , HL_c , LH_c and HH_c : First level DWT coefficients for cover image
LL_{c1} , HL_{c1} , LH_{c1} and HH_{c1}: Second level DWT coefficients for cover image

STEP 2: Read the Images
M_w$\leftarrow$ MRI.bmp (Cover image of size 512×512)

STEP 3: Perform DWT on Cover image
//Apply second level DWT on cover image
$[LL_c, HL_c, LH_c \text{ and } HH_c] \leftarrow$ DWT (M_w, wavelet filter);
$[LL_{c1}, HL_{c1}, LH_{c1} \text{ and } HH_{c1}] \leftarrow$ DWT (LL_c, wavelet filter);

STEP 4: Convert Watermarking text to Binary bits
// converting text watermark (JUIT) into binary bits
Wtxt $\leftarrow$ *binary(Text Watermark);*

STEP 5: Replace '(0,1)' by '(-1,1)' in the watermarking bits
// bit stream is transformed into a sequence w(1) w(2)....w(L) by replacing the 0 by
-1 and 1 by 1, L is the length of string
$-1 \leftarrow 0 \text{ and } 1 \leftarrow 1;$

STEP 6: Perform error correcting codes to the watermarking bits just obtained to get the final watermarking bits.

$Wb \leftarrow$ error correcting code (watermark bits)

STEP 7: Embedding the text watermark
// text watermark is embeds into HH_{c1} sub-band
for $\propto \leftarrow 0.01 : 0.1$
$f(x, y) = f(x, y)(1 + \propto \times Wb); f(x, y) \text{ and } f(x, y)$ is DWT coefficients before and after
embedding process
end;

STEP 8: Obtain the Watermarked Image W_d
//Apply Inverse DWT to LL_c , HL_c , LH_c and HH_c with modified and unmodified
DWT coefficients
$W_d \leftarrow$ *inverse DWT(LL_c, HL_c, LH_c and HH_c, wavelet filter);*
end:

5.4.4 Extraction Algorithm for Text Watermark

In the watermark extraction procedure, both the received image and the original
image are decomposed into the two levels. It is assumed that the original image is
available for the extraction process.

start:
STEP 1: Variable Declaration
Medical Image(MRI): cover image
C_w: read the cover image
α : scale factor
DWT : discrete wavelet transforms
Wavelet filters: Haar

LL_c , HL_c , LH_c and HH_c : First level DWT coefficients for cover image
LL_{c1} , HL_{c1} , LH_{c1} and HH_{c1}: Second level DWT coefficients for cover image

start:
STEP 2: Perform DWT on Watermarked image (possibly distorted)
// original image is also available for extraction process
$[LL_c, HL_c, LH_c$ and $HH_c,$ *wavelet filter*]$\leftarrow$ DWT (W_d, wavelet filter);

STEP 3: Watermark extraction

$$W_r b = \frac{\left(f_r^{'}(x,y) - f(x,y)\right)}{\alpha f(x,y)} ; f_r^{'}(x, y) \; are \; \text{the DWT coefficients of the received image.}$$

//finally extracted watermark taken as sign(either positive or negative)
$W_e b \leftarrow$ positive or negative sign(W_rb);

STEP 4: Perform error correcting codes to $W_e b$
// also modify the watermarking bits by replacing '(-1,1)' by '(0,1)' to get the final
watermark.

$$W_f b \leftarrow \text{error correcting code} \left(W_e b \right)$$

STEP 5: Convert the watermark bits into text to get the original watermark

Original text $\leftarrow$ convert (watermark bits)
end:

5.5   Experimental Results and Performance Analysis

In this section, the performance of combined ECCs-DWT-SVD watermarking algorithm is described. The gray–level medical image of size 512×512 [20] is used as
the cover image. Figure 5.2a show the MRI cover image and Fig. 5.2b–d show the
watermarked image at different gain. Figure 5.3a, b show the Lena image as image
watermark and the patient's identity/reference "*Amit_BXBPS4951D_MR19*" as text

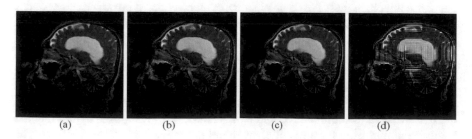

(a)   (b)   (c)   (d)

Fig. 5.2 Original and watermarked MRI images (**a**) original image and watermarked images at
gain factor (**b**) 0.01 (**c**) 0.05 and (**d**) 0.5

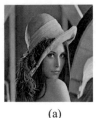

Patient's name_Patient's identity_Image code:
Amit_BXBPS4951D_MR19

(a)   (b)

Fig. 5.3 EPR data as (**a**) image and (**b**) text watermark

watermark respectively. The image watermark embedding method is based on DWT and SVD. However, the text watermark embedding method is based on encoding the text watermark using Hamming, BCH, Reed-Solomon and the hybrid code consisting of BCH and repetition code ECCs. The text watermark represented in 7-bit ASCII is embedded in five different ways for performance evaluation: first without ECC and next using four aforesaid ECCs. In the text watermarking process without using ECC, the text watermark size is 20 characters which is equivalent to 140 bits when represented in 7-bit ASCII. On using Hamming coded watermark the text watermark length becomes 245 bits. However, the encoded watermark length for BCH and Reed-Solomon error correction codes is 300 bits.

With repetition ECC, each original signal of a watermark is repeated N times in a block section, which is named as (N, 1). In this work, N is taken to be 3. The proposed hybrid method for multiple watermarking is implemented in MATLAB. The performance of proposed method is evaluated in terms of robustness against seven known signal processing attacks namely JPEG Compression, Median filtering, Gaussian low pass filter (LPF), sharpening mask, scaling Gaussian noise, salt & pepper noise and histogram equalization. The PSNR is used to measure the quality of the watermarked image. However, robustness of the extracted image and text watermarks are measured by NC and BER respectively. Also, the effect of the ECCs on BER is evaluated and compared for different watermark sizes. In the experiments, the gain factor (α) is taken from 0.01 to 0.1. The values of PSNR, NC and BER so obtained are illustrated in Tables 5.1, 5.2, 5.3, 5.4, 5.5, and 5.6. Table 5.7 shows the superior performance of hybrid code over the other three ECCs. Without any noise attack, highest PSNR obtained with all considered error correcting codes (140 text bits) is 37.22 dB at $\alpha = 0.01$ whereas NC = 1 and BER = 0 at all chosen gain factors. It is verified that larger the gain factor, stronger is the robustness and smaller the gain factor, better is the image quality. Table 5.1 shows the performance (determined PSNR, NC and BER values) of the proposed hybrid method using Hamming ECC for text watermark size from 28 bits to 140 bits. The maximum NC value is 0.9951 at $\alpha = 0.05$ for the text watermark size = 140 bits. Table 5.2 shows the performance (determined NC and BER values) of the proposed hybrid method using Hamming ECC for nine different signal processing attacks at $\alpha = 0.05$. The highest NC value = 0.9949 is obtained against JPEG compression (quality factor = 100). However, the lowest NC value is 0.3011 against Salt and pepper attack with

Table 5.1 The effect of Hamming code on PSNR, NC and BER at different gain factor (α)

Gain (α)	1st level DWT decomposition					1st level DWT decomposition					2nd level DWT decomposition				
	PSNR value at different size of text watermark (bits)					NC value for image watermark at different size of text watermark (bits)					BER value for text watermark at different size of text watermark (bits)				
	28	56	84	112	140	28	56	84	112	140	28	56	84	112	140
0.01	40.93	39.22	38.34	37.72	37.22	0.8761	0.9043	0.9067	0.8921	0.8739	0	0	0	0	0
0.03	39.16	37.95	37.27	36.78	36.38	0.9890	0.9920	0.9927	0.9911	0.9881	0	0	0	0	0
0.05	35.89	35.28	34.89	34.61	34.36	0.9933	0.9948	0.9957	0.9958	0.9951	0	0	0	0	0
0.07	33.07	32.74	32.52	32.35	32.21	0.9923	0.9933	0.9937	0.9940	0.9938	0	0	0	0	0
0.09	30.82	30.61	30.48	30.37	30.28	0.9928	0.9933	0.9936	0.9939	0.9938	0	0	0	0	0
0.1	29.85	29.69	29.58	29.49	29.58	0.9929	0.9933	0.9934	0.9936	0.9934	0	0	0	0	0

Table 5.2 The effect of Hamming code on NC and BER against different attacks at gain factor (α) = 0.05

Attacks	Using Hamming code		Without using Hamming code	
	Image watermark (NC value)	Text watermark (BER value)	Image watermark (NC value)	Text watermark (BER value)
JPEG compression (QF = 100)	0.9950	0	0.9955	0
JPEG compression (QF = 60)	0.9325	0	0.9528	0
JPEG compression (QF = 20)	0.9653	0	0.9582	0
Sharpening mask (threshold = 0.1,0.3,0.5,0.7 and 0.9)	0.6073,0.6257, 0.6390,0.6486 and 0.6556	0	0.6338, 0.6507, 0.6630, 0.6711 and 0.6769	0
Median filtering [2 2] and [3 3]	0.9116 and 0.8885	0	0.9077 and 0.8856	0.7143 and 0
Scaling factor 2	0.7075	0	0.7172	0.7143
Scaling factor 2.5	0.6500	1.0126	0.659	1.4286
Gaussian LPF (standard deviation = 0.6)	0.8780	0	0.8672	0
Gaussian noise (Mean = 0, Var = 0.001)	0.7012	0	0.7101	0
Gaussian noise (Mean = 0, Var = 0.05)	0.3150	8.5714	0.3264	10
Salt & pepper noise with (Density = 0.001)	0.7553	0	0.7880	0
Salt & pepper noise with (Density = 0.1)	0.3011	0	0.3083	0.7143
Histogram equalization	0.5880	1.4286	0.5931	2.1429
Cropping attack	0.7451	4.5714	0.7173	5

Table 5.3 The effect of BCH code on PSNR, NC and BER at different gain factors

Gain factor (α)	1st level DWT decomposition					1st level DWT decomposition					2nd level DWT decomposition				
	PSNR value at different size of text watermark (bits)					NC value for image watermark at size of text watermark (bits)					BER value for text watermark at different size of text watermark (bits)				
	28	56	84	112	140	28	56	84	112	140	28	56	84	112	140
0.01	40.41	38.79	37.88	37.29	36.85	0.8759	0.8989	0.8893	0.8607	0.8393	0	0	0	0	0
0.03	38.81	37.62	36.91	36.44	36.07	0.9884	0.9909	0.9905	0.9864	0.9827	0	0	0	0	0
0.05	35.72	35.09	34.69	34.39	34.16	0.9938	0.9954	0.9957	0.9950	0.9940	0	0	0	0	0
0.07	32.98	32.64	32.39	32.22	32.08	0.9927	0.9937	0.9940	0.9939	0.9934	0	0	0	0	0
0.09	30.76	30.55	30.40	30.29	30.20	0.9929	0.9934	0.9938	0.9938	0.9936	0	0	0	0	0
0.1	29.81	29.64	29.52	29.43	29.35	0.9930	0.9934	0.9935	0.9935	0.9934	0	0	0	0	0

Table 5.4 The effect of BCH code on NC and BER against different attacks at gain factor $(\alpha) = 0.05$

Attacks	Using BCH code		Without using BCH code	
	NC value for image watermark	BER value for text watermark	NC value for image watermark	BER value for Text watermark
JPEG compression (QF = 100)	0.9942	0	0.9955	0
JPEG compression (QF = 60)	0.9234	0	0.9528	0
JPEG compression (QF = 20)	0.9723	0	0.9676	0
Sharpening mask with threshold = 0.1,0.3,0.5, 0.7 and 0.9	0.5986, 0.6161, 0.6293, 0.6388 and 0.6457	0	0.6338,0.6507, 0.6630,0.6711 and 0.6769	0
Median filtering [2 2] and [3 3]	0.9144 and 0.8896	0	0.9077, 0.8856	0.7143 and 0
Scaling factor 2	0.699	0	0.7172	0.7143
Scaling factor 2.5	0.646	0.7112	0.659	1.4286
Gaussian LPF (standard deviation = 0.6)	0.8612	0	0.8672	0
Gaussian noise with mean = 0, Var = 0.001	0.7063	0	0.7121	0
Gaussian noise (mean = 0, Var = 0.05)	0.3284	6.2843	0.3264	10
Salt & pepper noise (density = 0.001)	0.7825	0	0.7880	0
Salt & pepper noise (density = 0.1)	0.3086	0	0.3083	0.7143
Histogram equalization	0.585	0.7143	0.5931	2.1429
Cropping attack	0.7449	3.5714	0.7173	5

Table 5.5 The effect of Reed-Solomon code on PSNR, NC and BER at different gain factor

Gain (α)	1st level DWT decomposition PSNR value at different size of text watermark (bits)					1st level DWT decomposition NC value for image watermark at different size of text watermark (bits)					2nd level DWT decomposition BER value for text watermark at different size of text watermark (bits)				
	28	56	84	112	140	28	56	84	112	140	28	56	84	112	140
0.01	40.41	38.79	37.88	37.29	36.85	0.8759	0.893	0.8887	0.8784	0.8472	0	0	0	0	0
0.03	38.81	37.62	36.91	36.44	36.07	0.9888	0.9907	0.9902	0.9882	0.9833	0	0	0	0	0
0.05	35.72	35.09	34.69	34.39	34.16	0.9936	0.9950	0.9955	0.9957	0.9943	0	0	0	0	0
0.07	32.98	32.64	32.39	32.23	31.34	0.9926	0.9935	0.9939	0.9940	0.9938	0	0	0	0	0
0.09	30.76	30.55	30.40	30.29	29.70	0.9928	0.9934	0.9940	0.9939	0.9938	0	0	0	0	0
0.1	29.80	29.64	29.52	30.09	29.35	0.9930	0.9934	0.9936	0.9936	0.9933	0	0	0	0	0

Table 5.6 The effect of Reed-Solomon code on NC and BER against different attacks at gain factor $(\alpha) = 0.05$

	Using Reed-Solomon code		Without using Reed-Solomon code	
Attacks	NC value for image watermark	BER value for text watermark	NC value for image watermark	BER value for text watermark
JPEG compression (QF = 100)	0.9939	0	0.9955	0
JPEG compression (QF = 60)	0.9251	0	0.9528	0
JPEG compression (QF = 20)	0.9665	0	0.9676	0
Sharpening mask (threshold = 0.1,0.3,0.5, 0.7 and 0.9)	0.6028,0.6207, 0.6338,0.6431 and 0.6500	0	0.6338,0.6507,0.6630, 0.6711 and 0.6769	0
Median filtering [2 2] and [3 3]	0.9143 and 0.8896	0	0.9077, 0.8856	0.7143 and 0
Scaling factor 2	0.7008	0	0.7172	0.7143
Scaling factor 2.5	0.6444	0	0.659	1.4286
Gaussian LPF	0.8612	0	0.8872	0
Gaussian noise (mean = 0,Var = 0.001)	0.7011	0	0.7121	0
Gaussian noise (mean = 0,Var = 0.05)	0.3141	6.1321	0.3264	10
Salt & pepper noise with (density = 0.001)	0.7897	0	0.7880	0
Salt & pepper noise with (density = 0.1)	0.3085	0	0.3083	0.7143
Histogram equalization	0.5833	0.6693	0.5931	2.1429
Cropping attack	0.7453	3.5022	0.7173	5

Table 5.7 Hybrid code performance under PSNR, NC and BER at different gain factors

Gain factor (α)	1st level DWT decomposition			1st level DWT decomposition			2nd level DWT decomposition		
	PSNR value at different size of text watermark (bits)			NC value for image watermark at size of text watermark (bits)			BER value for text watermark at different size of text watermark (bits)		
	28	84	140	28	84	140	28	84	140
0.01	37.87	35.75	35	0.8994	0.755	0.6921	0	0	0
0.05	34.68	33.54	33.07	0.9961	0.9876	0.9814	0	0	0
0.09	30.4	29.93	29.73	0.994	0.9922	0.9905	0	0	0
0.1	29.51	29.13	28.96	0.9936	0.9924	0.9912	0	0	0

noise density equal to 0.1. The highest BER is obtained as 8.5714 against the Gaussian noise which is 10 for text watermarking without using Hamming code. Table 5.3 shows the performance (determined PSNR, NC and BER values) of the proposed hybrid method using BCH ECC for text watermark size from 28 bits to 140 bits. The maximum PSNR value is 36.85 dB at gain factor (α) = 0.05. However, the maximum NC value is 0.9940 at α = 0.05 for the text watermark size = 140 bits. Table 5.4 shows performance (determined NC and BER values) of the proposed hybrid method using BCH ECC for nine different signal processing attacks at α = 0.05. The highest NC value = 0.9942 is obtained against JPEG compression (quality factor = 100). However, the lowest NC is 0.3086 against salt and pepper attack with density 0.1. The highest BER have been found 6.284 against Gaussian noise which is 10 for text watermarking without applying BCH code.

Table 5.5 shows the performance (determined PSNR, NC and BER values) of the proposed hybrid method using Reed-Solomon ECC for text watermark size from 28 bits to 140 bits. The maximum PSNR value is 36.85 dB at α = 0.05. However, the maximum NC value is 0.9943 at α = 0.05 for the text watermark size = 140 bits. Table 5.6 shows performance (determined NC and BER values) of the proposed hybrid method using Reed-Solomon ECC for nine different signal processing attacks at α = 0.05. The highest NC value = 0.9939 is obtained against JPEG compression (quality factor = 100). However, the lowest NC value is 0.3085 against Salt and pepper noise with density 0.1. The highest BER have been found 6.1321 against Gaussian noise which is 10 for text watermarking without Reed-Solomon code. Table 5.7 shows the performance (determined PSNR, NC and BER values) of the proposed hybrid method using hybrid ECC for text watermark size from 28 bits to 140 bits. The maximum PSNR value is 35 dB at gain factor (α) = 0.01. However, the maximum NC value is 0.9912 at α = 0.1 for the text watermark size = 140 bits.

Table 5.8 shows the performance (determined NC and BER values) comparison of hybrid error correcting with the other three error correcting codes. During analysis only those attacks are considered where the BER values are not zero. It is observed that the maximum NC value with hybrid error correcting coding method is obtained as 0.9481 against 0.7451, 0.7173 and 0.7451 as obtained by Hamming,

Table 5.8 Performance comparison of different ECCs against signal processing attacks at gain factor (α) = 0.05

Attacks	Using Hamming code		Using BCH code		Using Reed-Solomon code		Using Hybrid coding	
	Image watermark (NC value)	Text watermark (BER value)	Image watermark (NC value)	Text watermark (BER value)	Image watermark (NC value)	Text watermark (BER value)	Image watermark (NC value)	Text watermark (BER value)
Scaling factor 2.5	0.65	1.0126	0.659	1.4286	0.65	1.0126	0.692	0.3214
Gaussian noise (mean = 0, Var = 0.05)	0.315	8.5714	0.3264	10	0.315	8.5714	0.3289	2.618
Salt & pepper noise (density = 0.1)	0.3011	0	0.3083	0.7143	0.3011	0	0.3232	0
Histogram equalization	0.588	1.4286	0.5931	2.1429	0.588	1.4286	0.8187	0
Cropping attack	0.7451	4.5714	0.7173	5	0.7451	4.5714	0.9481	1.666

Table 5.9 Effect of cover images on PSNR, NC and BER values using hybrid error correcting code at gain factor (α) = 0.05

Image Type	PSNR (dB)	NC Value	BER Value
MRI	28.45	0.9475	0
CT Scan	29.21	0.9227	0
Ultrasound	32.45	0.9657	0
Barbara	25.87	0.9879	0

Table 5.10 Comparison of NC values with other reported methods

Attacks	Tripathi et al. [6]	Mahajan and Patil [8]	With Hybrid coding
Scaling (scaling factor = 0.5 and 1.5)	0.3137 and 0.7031	Not reported	0.3922 and 0.831
Rotation (350 degree)	0.7478	0.1413	0.8690
JPEG compression (QF = 20)	0.9586	Not reported	0.9723
Salt & pepper noise	Not reported	-0.0013	0.3232
Cropping	Not reported	0.1411	0.9481

BCH and Reed-Solomon error correcting code respectively. The maximum BER value is obtained with the hybrid ECC method is 2.618 against Gaussian Noise (Mean = 0, Var-0.05). However, the BER value is obtained with Hamming, BCH and Reed-Solomon error correcting codes are 8.5714, 10 and 8.5714, respectively.

Overall, the hybrid proposed method is better than the other three error correcting codes. The performance of proposed method was also determined with four different cover images i.e. MRI, CT Scan, Ultrasound and Barbara images. Table 5.9 shows the PSNR, NC and BER values obtained by the proposed method with these cover images at gain factor (α) = 0.05. The highest PSNR 32.45 dB and NC value 0.9879 is obtained with Ultrasound and Barbara image respectively. For both of these images, the BER obtained is zero. The performance of the proposed hybrid method with the hybrid ECC is compared with the method proposed in [6] and [8] for five different attacks. The results are shown in Table 5.10. It is observed that the hybrid method gives better performance in terms of robustness than other reported methods [6, 8].

Figure 5.4 shows the comparison between four ECCs in terms of NC values against known attacks using size of the text watermark = 140 bits. Referring this figure it is observed that the maximum NC value with hybrid ECC is obtained as 0.9481 against the cropping attack. However, with the Hamming, the BCH and the Reed-Solomon error correcting code is obtained as 0.7451, 0.7173 and 0.7451 respectively. The minimum NC value with hybrid code is obtained as 0.3232 against the Salt & Pepper Noise with density = 0.1. However, with the Hamming, the BCH and the Reed-Solomon ECC is obtained as 0.3011, 0.3083 and 0.3011 respectively. Figure 5.5 shows the comparison between four ECCs in terms of BER values against known attacks using size of the text watermark = 140 bits. In this figure, it is observed that the maximum and minimum BER value with hybrid code is obtained

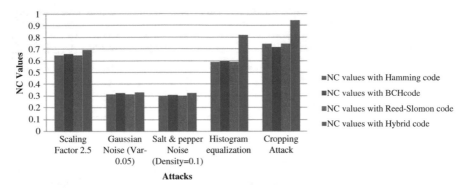

Fig. 5.4 NC performance with different ECCs against known attacks at gain factor (α) = 0.05

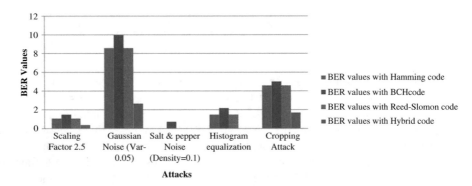

Fig. 5.5 BER performance with different ECCs against known attacks at gain factor (α) = 0.05

as 2.618 and zero against the Gaussian Noise (Mean = 0, Var = 0.05) and Salt & pepper noise respectively. However, the maximum BER value with the Hamming, the BCH and the Reed-Solomon error correcting code are obtained as 8.5714, 10 and 8.5714, respectively.

Figures 5.6 and 5.7 show the PSNR and NC values obtained by the proposed method with the hybrid ECC against different cover images respectively at the gain factor α = 0.05. In Fig. 5.6, the maximum PSNR value 32.45 dB has been obtained with Ultrasound image. However, the minimum PSNR value is 25.87 dB is obtained with the Barbara image. In Fig. 5.7, the highest NC value has been obtained as 0.9879 with Barbara image with the minimum NC value of 0.9227 with the CT Scan image.

Fig. 5.6 PSNR performance of the proposed method for different cover images using hybrid error correcting code at gain factor (α) = 0.05

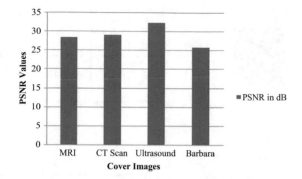

Fig. 5.7 NC performance of the proposed method for different cover images using hybrid error correcting code at gain factor (α) = 0.05

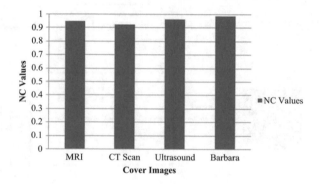

5.5.1   Performance Evaluation of the Proposed Method Using Encryption

In order to enhance the security of the text watermark, encryption is applied to the ASCII representation of the text watermark before encoding and embedding. Figure 5.8 shows the encryption based watermark embedding and extraction process. The strength of watermark is tested by varying the gain factor in the watermarking algorithm. For testing the robustness and quality of the watermarked image, the proposed scheme was implemented in MATLAB. The robustness of the image and text watermarks is evaluated by determining NC and BER respectively.

The quality of the watermarked image is evaluated by PSNR. Figure 5.9a shows the MRI cover image and Figs. 5.9b–d show watermarked images at different gain factors 0.01, 0.05 and 0.5, respectively. The text watermark is the patient data as shown in Fig. 5.10. In the experiment, values of PSNR, NC and BER are illustrated in Table 5.11 to Table 5.13 for varying gain factor (α) in the range from 0.01 to 0.5. However, it is observed that the overall performance of the proposed method depends on the size of the watermarks, gain factor and the noise variation.

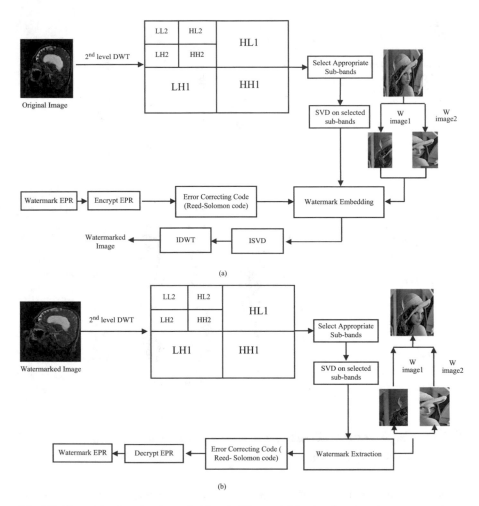

Fig. 5.8 Encryption based watermark (**a**) embedding and (**b**) extraction process

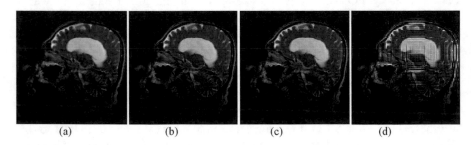

Fig. 5.9 Original and watermarked MRI images (**a**) original image and watermarked images with gain factor; (**b**) 0.01; (**c**) 0.05 and (**d**) 0.5

Patient's name_Patient's ID_Image code_Blood group_Date of birth_Doctor name
_Doctor ID_Patient's report_Hospital address:
AKSingh_BXBPS4951D_ICT196/B+/20 05
_79_DrMDave_506516441444_StrokeAmennea01Aug2014_Departmentof
ComputerEngineeringNIT

Fig. 5.10 EPR data as text watermark

Table 5.11 shows effect of gain factor on performance (determined PSNR, NC and BER values) of the proposed method for different size of watermark without any noise attack. With the encryption and ECC, maximum PSNR value is 28.17 dB and BER = 0 against maximum size of watermark at gain factor (α) = 0.01. Here, the NC value is smallest of all the obtained values at this gain factor. However, the maximum NC value is 0.9697 at α = 0.1. With the encryption and without ECC, the maximum PSNR obtained is 28.7 dB at gain factor (α) = 0.01. The maximum NC and BER values are obtained for α = 0.1 and 0.5 respectively. It is observed that larger gain factor results in stronger robustness of the extracted watermark whereas smaller gain factor provides better PSNR.

Table 5.12 shows the performance (determined NC and BER values) of the proposed watermarking method for eight different attacks. The highest BER value of 7.1429 has been obtained against Scaling attack (with scaling factor = 2) with encryption and ECC which is slightly better than the BER performance with encryption and without ECC (BER = 10.9606). Table 5.13 shows the performance (PSNR, NC value and BER) of the proposed method for different cover images. The highest BER and PSNR were obtained with Ultrasound image at gain factor (α) = 0.05. The NC and BER values obtained by the proposed method for image and text watermarks with those reported by Singh et al. [7] for nine different attack categories are compared in Table 5.14. Figure 5.11 show the comparion under NC performance with other reported technique [7].

The following observation are apparent for the proposed method:

(i) *Higher embedding capacity*: The size of text watermark is 20 characters for the method proposed Singh et al. [7]. However, proposed method can embed 116 characters with acceptable PSNR.
(ii) *Improved performance*: As inferred from Table 5.14, the maximum NC value with the proposed method is 0.9956 against 0.9939 obtained by the method proposed by Singh et al. [7]. However, the maximum BER of the proposed method is only 2.039 as against 6.1321 obtained by Singh et al. in [7].
(iii) *Enhanced security*: Security of the text watermark is enhanced by applying encryption method on the text watermark before embedding in to the medical comer image.

Overall, the proposed method is better in terms of robustness, security and capacity to that of the method proposed in [7]. The robustness (determined NC values) of the image watermark is also tested with 'Checkmark' benchmarking software [21, 22].

Table 5.11 Effect of gain factor on PSNR, NC and BER performance with varying text watermark sizes

| Gain (α) | With Encryption and ECC | | | | | | With Encryption and Without ECC | | | | | |
| | 116 characters | | | 60 characters | | | 116 characters | | | 60 characters | | |
	PSNR (dB)	NC Value	BER	PSNR (dB)	NC Value	BER	PSNR (dB)	NC Value	BER	PSNR (dB)	NC Value	BER
0.01	28.17	0.5247	0	28.61	0.6065	0	28.7	0.6075	0	29.37	0.6976	0
0.05	28.02	0.9288	0	28.45	0.9432	0	28.54	0.9479	0	29.18	0.9572	0
0.09	27.17	0.9668	0	27.52	0.9726	0	27.59	0.9734	0	28.09	0.9772	0
0.1	26.85	0.9697	0	27.17	0.9746	0	27.24	0.9745	0	27.7	0.9771	0
0.5	15.39	0.9179	0	15.42	0.9185	0	15.42	0.9188	1.1084	15.45	0.9195	1.6667

Table 5.12 Effect of encryption and ECC on NC and BER against different attacks at gain factor (α) = 0.05

Attacks	With encryption and Reed-Solomon coding		With encryption and without Reed-Solomon coding	
	NC value for image watermark	BER value for text watermark	NC value for image watermark	BER value for text watermark
JPEG compression (QF = 100)	0.9253	0	0.945	0
JPEG compression (QF = 60)	0.7603	0	0.8034	0
JPEG compression (QF = 20)	0.8261	0.1232	0.8104	4.4335
Sharpening mask (threshold = 0.1,0.5 and 0.9)	0.6137,0.6299, 0.6409	0	0.6236,0.6395, 0.6491	0,0.1232, 0.1232
Median filtering [1 1], [2 2] and [3 3]	0.9257, 0.7968, 0.7329	0, 1.4778,0	0.9450, 0.7784, 0.7297	0, 4.5567, 2.8325
Scaling factor 1	0.9257	0	0.945	0
Scaling factor 2	0.7533	7.1429	0.7625	10.9606
Gaussian LPF (standard deviation = 0.5)	0.9257	0	0.945	0
Gaussian noise (Mean = 0, Var = 0.001)	0.8601	0	0.8748	0
Gaussian noise (Mean = 0, Var = 0.01)	0.7194	1.3547	0.721	4.2512
Salt & pepper noise (density = 0.001)	0.8009	0	0.8147	0.1232
Salt & pepper noise (density = 0.1)	0.5322	0.8621	0.5965	1.327
Histogram equalization	0.7974	0	0.8221	0

Table 5.13 Effect of cover image on PSNR, NC and BER at gain factor (α) = 0.05

Cover image	With encryption		
	PSNR (dB)	NC value	BER
Brain	30.82	0.9565	0
CT Scan	28.02	0.9257	0
Ultrasound	32.36	0.9667	8.2512
MRI	28.02	0.9288	0
Barbara	24.27	0.9664	0

Table 5.14 Comparison of NC and BER values with other reported method

Attacks	Singh et al. [7] with watermark size = 20 character		Proposed method with watermark size = 20 character	
	NC value for image watermark	BER value for text watermark	NC value for image watermark	BER value for text watermark
JPEG compression (QF = 100)	0.9939	0	0.9956	0
JPEG compression (QF = 60)	0.9251	0	0.9318	0
JPEG compression (QF = 20)	0.9665	0	0.9676	0
Sharpening mask (threshold = 0.9)	0.65	0	0.7211	0
Median filtering [2 2] and [3 3]	0.9143 and 0.8896	0	0.9259 and 0.8910	0
Scaling factor 2	0.7008	0	0.8013	0
Gaussian LPF	0.8612	0	0.9943	0
Gaussian noise (Mean = 0, Var = 0.001)	0.7011	0	0.7227	0
Gaussian noise (mean = 0,Var-0.05)	0.3141	6.1321	0.421	2.039
Salt & pepper noise (density = 0.001)	0.7897	0	0.7936	0
Salt & pepper noise (density = 0.1)	0.3085	0	0.3214	0
Histogram equalization	0.5833	0.6693	0.5841	0.1429
Cropping attack	0.7453	3.5022	0.7465	1.7143

In Table 5.15, the maximum NC value of the extracted watermark under different attacks is shown at gain factor = 0.05. The maximum NC value of 0.8753 is obtained by the proposed method against the Scale attack. However, the minimum NC value is 0.5102 against the Collage attack. In this table, all the NC values are acceptable except the Collage attack which is less than 0.7. Figure 5.12 gives graphical representation of the robustness performance of the proposed method against 'Checkmark' attacks.

From the above extensive discussion, we have observed that the experimental results for robustness (i.e. NC and BER values) of image and text watermark taking five different attacks and considering the four ECC encodings are shown in Table 5.8. With reference to Table 5.8 it can be inferred that the NC values vary in the range from 0.3011 to 0.9481 at gain factor 'α' = 0.05. The best performance in terms of robustness is obtained in case of hybrid ECC encoding where the NC value is highest for each attack compared to other encoding methods under same attacks.

Fig. 5.11 Comparison of proposed method with existing technique for Checkmark Attacks

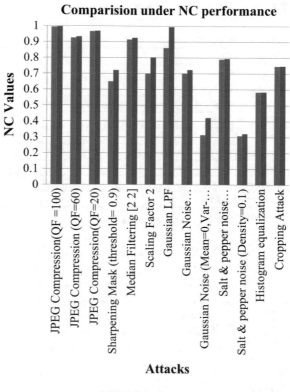

The highest NC value obtained is 0.9481 for the cropping attack with hybrid ECC encoding. Therefore, it can be concluded that the suggested embedding algorithm offers best robustness with hybrid ECC encoding along with acceptable perceptual quality of the watermarked image (PSNR > 28dB) without attacks. Further, from Table 5.8, it is evident that lowest bit error rate (BER) for all attacks is obtained for hybrid ECC encoding of text watermark and up to 39.23% enhancement in NC value for image watermark is achieved. From Table 5.10, it can be concluded that the proposed algorithm offers up to six times enhancement in NC value as compared to the other reported techniques [6, 8]. In addition, the performance of the proposed algorithm was evaluated after encrypting and then encoding the text watermark using Reed-Solomon ECC. The proposed method offered up to six times enhancement in embedding capacity, 15.45% enhancement in robustness and 3% reduced BER over the other reported method [7]. In addition, the proposed method provides extra level of security of the text watermark by encrypting it before embedding.

Table 5.15 Effect of 'Checkmark' attacks at gain factor (α) = 0.05

'Checkmark' attacks	Maximum NC values for image watermark
Collage	0.5102
Template remove	0.7222
Rows and columns removal	*0.7284*
Denoising followed by perceptual remodulation (DPR)	0.7288
DPR_Corr attack	0.7255
Scale	0.8753
Trimmed mean	0.8696
Cropping	0.7862
Gaussian	0.7857
Hard thresholding	0.7164
Soft thresholding	0.8081
JPEG compression	0.723
Wavelet compression	0.7284
Medium filter	0.821
Mid point	0.7236
Projective	0.8235
Ratio	0.7284
Rotation/scaling	0.7284
Stirmark	0.7284
Shearing	0.7284
Warp	0.7284
Wiener	0.7255

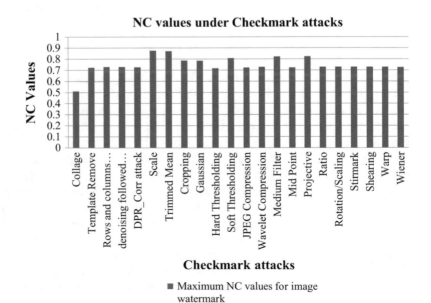

Fig. 5.12 NC performance of the proposed method against 'Checkmark' attacks

Further, the NC values under different attacks using benchmark software 'Checkmark' are shown in Table 5.15 from which it is found that the suggested technique is robust against the 'Checkmark' attacks except the NC value for Collage attack where NC value is less than 0.7.

5.6 Summary

In this chapter, we have presented a robust hybrid multiple watermarking technique in wavelet domain using Hamming, BCH, Reed-Solomon and the hybrid ECC code for encoding the text watermark before embedding along with direct embedding of image watermark using DWT and SVD. It is observed that the watermarking method based on hybrid ECC code has better performance as compared to the other three ECCs. Further, the robustness, security and capacity of the multiple watermarks (image and text) are enhanced by encrypting the text watermark followed by encoding it using Reed-Solomon ECC. The maximum NC and BER value of the encryption based watermarking method using ECC has been obtained against the Gaussian LPF and the scaling attack, respectively. However, the performance of method depends on the watermark size, gain factor and the noise variations. In addition, to make the data an error correctable, additional bit in the form of ECC is required to be added in the original bits. However, to further improve the error correction capability the length of the error correction code may be suitably increased. The main contributions of this chapter are identified as follows:

(i) The proposed hybrid technique using DWT and SVD improves the robustness and imperceptibility as compared to DWT and SVD applied individually.
(ii) For the identity authentication purpose, two watermarks (text and image) are embedded into the cover image instead of single watermark, which provides extra level of security. This has superior performance in applications such as telemedicine and tele-diagnosis. In the proposed method, two watermarks are embedded simultaneously.
(iii) The proposed hybrid method maximum NC value with hybrid error correcting coding offered significant enhancements in robustness over the other three error correction codes. Further, the robustness performance of the proposed method is better than other existing techniques. However, the proposed encryption based multiple watermarking method offers significant improvements in embedding capacity, robustness and reduced BER over the other existing techniques.
(iv) Futher, the first level decomposition in DWT has been used for embedding the image watermark. This gives advantages like maximizing the watermark embedding area. The first level decomposition leads to improved texture in the extracted watermark image with better imperceptibility.

References

1. A.K. Singh, M. Dave, A. Mohan, Robust and secure multiple watermarking in wavelet domain. A special issue on advanced signal processing technologies and systems for healthcare applications (ASPTSHA). J. Med. Imaging Health Inf. **5**(2), 406–414 (2015)
2. A.K. Singh, B. Kumar, M. Dave, A. Mohan, Robust and imperceptible dual watermarking for telemedicine applications. Wirel. Pers. Commun. **80**(4), 1415–1433 (2014)
3. A. Sharma, A.K. Singh, S.P. Ghrera, Robust and secure multiple watermarking technique for medical images. Wirel. Pers. Commun. **92**(4), 1611–1624 (2017)
4. A.K. Singh, M. Dave, A. Mohan, Hybrid technique for robust and imperceptible multiple watermarking using medical images. J. Multimedia Tools Appl. **75**(14), 8381–8401 (2015)
5. R. Dhanalakshmi, K. Thaiyalnayaki, Dual watermarking scheme with encryption. Int. J. Comput. Sci. Inf. Security **7**(1), 248–253 (2010)
6. S. Tripathi, N. Ramesh, A. Bernito, K.J. Neeraj, A DWT based dual image watermarking technique for authenticity and watermark protection. Signal Image Process. Int. J. (SIPIJ) **1**(2), 33–45 (2010)
7. A.K. Singh, M. Dave, A. Mohan, Hybrid technique for robust and imperceptible dual watermarking using error correcting codes for application in telemedicine. Int. J. Electron. Security Digit. Forensics **6**(4), 285–305 (2014)
8. L.H. Mahajan, S.A. Patil, Image watermarking scheme using SVD. Int. J. Adv. Res. Sci. Eng. **2**(6), 69–77 (2013)
9. C.-C. Lai, C.-C. Tsai, Digital image watermarking using discrete wavelet transform and singular value decomposition. IEEE Trans. Instrum. Meas. **59**(11), 3060–3063 (2010)
10. N. Terzjia, M. Repges, K. Luck, W. Geisselhardt, Digital image watermarking using discrete wavelet transform: performance comparison of error correction codes, in Proceedings of IASTED, 2002
11. B. Kumar, S. Bind, D.S. Chauhan, Wavelet based imperceptible medical image watermarking using spread-spectrum, in 37th International Conference on Telecommunications and Signal Processing, Berlin, Germany, pp. 660–664, 2014
12. A. Giakoumaki, S. Pavlopoulos, D. Koutsouris, Secure and efficient health data management through multiple watermarking on medical images. Med. Biol. Eng. Comput. **44**, 619–631 (2006)
13. C.-C. Chang, W.-L. Tai, C.-C. Lin, A multipurpose wavelet-based image watermarking, Proceedings of International Conference on Innovative Computing, Information and Control, pp. 70–73, 2006
14. A. Kannamma, K. Pavithra, S. Subha Rani, Double watermarking of dicom medical images using wavelet decomposition technique. Eur. J. Sci. Res. **70**, 46–55 (2012)
15. K. Wu, W. Yan, J. Du, A robust dual digital-image watermarking technique, in International Conference on Computational Intelligence and Security Workshop, pp. 668–671, 2007
16. C. Chemak, M.S. Bouhlel, J.C. Lapayre, A new scheme of robust image watermarking: the double watermarking algorithm, in Proceedings of the 2007 Summer Computer Simulation Conference, SCSC 2007, San Diego, CA, USA, pp. 1201–1208, 2007
17. H. Shen, B. Chen, From single watermark to dual watermark: a new approach for image watermarking. Comput. Electr. Eng. **38**, 1310–1324 (2012)
18. S. Zinger, Z. Jin, H. Maitre, Optimization of watermarking performances using error correcting codes and repetition, in Communications and Multimedia Security Issues of the New Century, pp. 229–240, 2001
19. W. Abdul, P. Carre, P. Gaborit, Error correcting codes for robust color wavelet watermarking. EURASIP J. Inf. Security **2013**(1), 1–17 (2013)
20. MedPixTM medical image database available at http://rad.usuhs.mil/medpix/medpix.html
21. http://watermarking.unige.ch/Checkmark/
22. S. Pereira, S. Voloshynovskiy, M. Madueño, S. Marchand-Maillet, T Pun, Second generation benchmarking and application oriented evaluation, in Proceeding of Information Hiding Workshop III, Pittsburgh, PA, USA, pp. 340–353, 2001

Chapter 6
Secure Spread Spectrum Based Multiple Watermarking Technique for Medical Images

Amit Kumar Singh, Basant Kumar, Ghanshyam Singh, and Anand Mohan

6.1 Introduction

The significant advancements in information and communication technologies (ICT) [1] has opened up newer opportunities for telemedicine by facilitating medical data transmission across geographical boundaries through Internet, mobile networks, and other wireless/wired communication channels and thus covering rural/remote areas, accident sites, ambulance, and hospitals. However, the transmission of medical data over an open communication channel poses different possibilities of threat that can severely affect its authenticity, integrity, and confidentiality [2]. Digital watermarking studies have always been driven by the improvement of robustness and a current security tool to protect electronic patient record (EPR) [3].

On the contrary, security has received little attention in the watermarking community. The first difficulty is that security and robustness are neighbouring concepts, which are

A.K. Singh (✉)
Department of Computer Science & Engineering, Jaypee University of Information Technology, Waknaghat, Solan, India
e-mail: amit_245singh@yahoo.com

B. Kumar
Department of Electronics and Communication Engineering, Motilal Nehru National Institute of Technology, Allahabad, India
e-mail: singhbasant@yahoo.com

G. Singh
Department of Electronics and Communication Engineering, Jaypee University of Information Technology, Waknaghat, Solan, India
e-mail: drghanshyam.singh@yahoo.com

A. Mohan
Department of Electronics Engineering, Indian Institute of Technology (BHU), Varanasi, India
e-mail: profanandmohan@gmail.com

© Springer International Publishing AG 2017
A.K. Singh et al. (eds.), *Medical Image Watermarking*, Multimedia Systems and Applications, DOI 10.1007/978-3-319-57699-2_6

hardly perceived as different. Security deals with intentional attacks whereas robustness is observed as degradation in data fidelity due to common signal processing operations. Also, digital watermarking may not be secure despite its robustness [4]. Therefore, security of the watermark becomes a critical issue in various applications. The problem of watermark security can be solved using spread-spectrum scheme [2, 5–10]. Spread-spectrum is a technique designed to be good at combating interference due to jamming, hiding of a signal by transmitting it at low power, and achieving secrecy. These properties make spread-spectrum very popular in present-day digital watermarking.

The subsequent section of the chapter is structured as follows: The related and recent state-of-the-art techniques are provided in Sect. 6.2. The main contribution of the work is summarized in Sect. 6.3. The spread-spectrum Watermark Design is reported in Sect. 6.4. Section 6.5 describes the proposed work. Experimental results and brief analysis of the work is reported in Sect. 6.6. Next, our summary of the chapter is presented in Sect. 6.7.

6.2 Related Work

Brief reviews of recent and related watermarking methods are presented as follows:

Recently, in [2] an image watermarking scheme based on spread-spectrum technique was proposed in which different watermark messages were hidden in the same transform coefficients of the cover image using uncorrelated codes, *i.e.* low cross correlation value (orthogonal/near orthogonal) among codes. The authors have also proposed another algorithm [5] based on spread-spectrum technique in which two different pseudo noise (PN sequence) vectors of size identical to the size of each sub-band column are generated for each watermark message bit. This algorithm further enhances the watermarking capacity in wavelet domain. The performance of the algorithm in [5] has been analysed for text watermark in [10]. These methods are robust and secure against known attacks. D-Ferrer and Sebe´ [11] proposed a spread spectrum based invertible watermarking method for image authentication purpose in lossless format. The method is robust and highly imperceptible. Das et al. [12] proposed a watermarking method based on spread spectrum technique. The method is designed from the analytical study of state transition behavior of non-group cellular automata and the basic cryptography/encryption scheme to provide the data authenticity and security. Multiple messages have been embedded using complimentary modulation function with M–ary modulation. The experimental results have shown that the method is robust against various signal processing attacks. Interleaving and interference cancellation methods are applied to improve the performance of the method as compared to conventional matched filter detection.

Basant et al. [2] proposed a secure spread-spectrum based watermarking algorithms for embedding sensitive medical information such as doctor signature and hospital logo into radiological image for identity authentication purposes. These watermarking schemes used watermarks in binary image format only. In this method, different watermark messages are hidden in the same transform coefficients of the cover image using PN code. Performance of the method has been analyzed by varying the gain factor, sub-band decomposition levels, size of watermarks, wavelet filters and medical image modalities. The simulation results have shown that the proposed method achieved higher security and robustness against JPEG attacks. Also, they proposed another algorithm [5] based on spread-spectrum technique in which, two different pseudo noise (PN sequence) vectors of size identical to the size of each sub-band column are generated for each watermark message bit. So, this algorithm enhanced the watermarking capacity when compared with previous algorithm as proposed in [2]. Performance of the spread-spectrum based watermarking algorithm [5] has been tested for text watermark in [10]. The algorithm is applied for embedding text file represented in binary arrays using ASCII code into host digital radiological image for potential telemedicine applications. In order to enhance the robustness of text watermarks like patient identity code, BCH (Bose, Ray-Chaudhuri, Hocquenghem) error correcting code (ECC) is applied to the ASCII representation of the text watermark before embedding. Robustness and performance of the scheme was tested against some known signal processing attacks like compression, filtering, channel noise, sharpening, and histogram equalization.

Singh et al. [13] presents a robust and secure digital watermarking scheme for its potential application in tele-medicine. The algorithm embeds different medical text watermarks into selected sub-band DWT coefficients of the cover medical image using spread-spectrum technique. In the embedding process, the cover image is decomposed up to third level DWT coefficients. Three different text watermarks are embedded into the selected horizontal and vertical sub band DWT coefficients of the first, second and third level

The medical image watermarking approaches in general have focused on achieving secure and bandwidth efficient transmission of medical data. Multiple watermarking of medical images aims to simultaneously embed various types of medical watermarks on the cover medical image addressing the issues of data security, data compaction, unauthorized access and temper proofing. The proposed multiple watermarking method attempts to simultaneously address these issues consisting of different characteristics and requirements which provide effective protection mechanism for the authenticity of patient identity in the application.

6.3   Main Contribution of the Work

The objective of this method is to provide a valuable solution for different health data management issues to involve hiding multiple watermarks within cover medical image and hidden watermarks can be later recovered at the receiver side for purposes of ownership verification and unique authentication. In order to presents a secure spread-spectrum based multiple watermarking method for medical images in wavelet transform domain. Two different watermarks in the form of image and text are embedding simultaneously into medical cover image. The algorithm uses pseudo-noise (PN) sequences of each image watermark bit, which are embedding column wise into the selected DWT sub-bands coefficients. The selection of the wavelet coefficients for embedding is done by thresholding the coefficient values present in that column. In the embedding process, the cover image is decomposed at second level DWT. The image and text watermark are embedded into the selective coefficients of the first level and second level DWT respectively. In order to enhance the robustness of text watermarks, an error correcting code is applied to the ASCII representation of the text watermark before embedding. The results are obtained by varying the gain factor, sub-band decomposition levels, size of watermark, and different cover images.

The performance of the proposed watermarking method is analyzed against known attacks. The method was found to be robust against such attacks. In addition, the performance of the proposed method has been extensively evaluated for the text watermark along with BCH code and encryption techniques which is presented in Sects. 6.1 and 6.6.2, respectively. The encoded/encrypted text watermark is then embedded at multiple levels of the DWT sub-bands. The performance of the methods are compared with other reported techniques and have been found to be giving superior performance in terms of robustness, imperceptibility, embedding capacity and security as suggested by other authors. Moreover, the performance of the multiple watermarking method is also tested with encryption and BCH error correction code simultaneously in Sect. 6.3. The encryption and BCH error correction code both are applying to the sensitive patient data/report before embedding in to the medical cover image to enhance the security and robustness of the text watermark respectively. The performance of the technique is extensively evaluated and experimental results demonstrated that the method is robust, higher imperceptible, large embedding capacity, and secure than other reported technique.

6.4 Spread-Spectrum Watermark Design

There are two components to build a strong watermark: the *watermark structure* and the *insertion strategy*. For a watermark to be robust and secure, these components must be designed correctly. This can be achieved by placing the watermark explicitly in the perceptually most significant components of the data. Once the significant components are located, Gaussian noise is injected therein. The choice of this distribution gives resilient performance against collusion attacks (the mixing of several watermarked versions of the same content). The Gaussian watermark also gives strong performance in the face of quantization [2].

Watermark Structure: In its most basic implementation, a watermark consists of a sequence of real numbers $X = x_1, x_2,.......x_n$. In practice, a watermark is created where each value x_i is chosen independently according to Gaussian distribution N $(0, 1)$, where $N (\mu, \sigma^2)$ denotes a normal distribution with mean μ and variance σ^2.

Watermarking Procedure: Extract from host digital document D, a sequence of values $V = v_1, v_2,......v_n$, into which a watermark $X = x_1, x_2,.......x_n$ is inserted to obtain an adjusted sequence of values $W = w_1, w_2,......,w_n$ and then insert it back into the host in place of V to obtain a watermarked document $(D*)$.

Inserting Watermark: When X is inserted into V to obtain W, a scaling parameter k is specified, which determines the extent to which X alters V. The method for computing W is

$$w_i = v_i + \propto x_i$$

The factor α can be viewed as a relative measure of embedding strength which is also known as gain factor (α). A large value of α will cause perceptual degradation in the watermarked document.

Choosing the Length 'n' of the Watermark: The choice of length n indicates the degree to which the watermark is spread out among the relevant components of the host image. In general, as the numbers of altered components are increased the extent to which they must be altered decreases.

Extracting and Evaluating the Similarity of Watermarks: It is highly unlikely that the extracted mark X^* will be identical to the original watermark X. Even the act of re-quantizing the watermarked document for delivery will cause X^* to deviate from X. The similarity of X and X^* is measured by

$$sim\left(X,X^*\right) = \frac{X^*.X}{\sqrt{X^*.X}} \qquad (6.1)$$

Many other measures are possible, including the standard correlation coefficient. To decide whether X and X^* match, one determines whether $sim(X, X^*) > T$, where T is some specified threshold. Setting the detection threshold is a classical decision estimation problem.

6.5   Proposed Method

For embedding medical text and image watermarks, a new DWT based spread-spectrum watermarking algorithm is proposed that uses medical image as cover. Dyadic sub-band decomposition is performed on the cover image using Haar wavelet transform. Table 6.1 shows the robustness requirement of EPR data at different sub-bands. This table indicates importance of the data according to robustness required. In the proposed method, the image watermark representing health centre name in binary image format is embedded into intermediate frequency sub-bands (HL1 and LH1) of the first level DWT coefficients and the patient's identity/reference as text watermark is embedded into selected sub-band DWT coefficients (HL2 and LH2) of the second level. The important allocation of watermarks according to robustness and capacity criteria at different sub-band is shown in Table 6.1.

The text watermark of eight characters representing patient identification code is converted into binary format using ASCII codes. In the embedding process, sub-band decomposition of the cover medical image is performed to obtain second level DWT coefficients. Different watermark bits are hidden in the same transform coefficients

Table 6.1 Allocation of watermarks according to robustness and capacity criteria at different sub-band

DWT sub-band	Capacity (embeddable coefficients)	Embedded watermark	
		EPR data	Robustness requirements
LH2	16384	Patient's identity/reference	High
HL2	16384	Patient's identity/reference	High
LH1	65356	Health center logo	Low

of the cover image using uncorrelated codes, i.e. low cross correlation value (orthogonal/near orthogonal) among codes. For each message (text and image) bit, two different pseudo noise (PN) sequence vectors of sizes identical to the size of DWT column vector are generated. A PN sequence is a sequence of binary numbers which appears to be random, but is in fact perfectly deterministic. The sequence appears to be random in the sense that the binary values and groups or runs of the same binary value occur in the sequence in the same proportion. PN sequences are a good tool for watermarking because of the following reasons [14]:

(i) PN sequence is having correlation properties, noise like characteristics and resistance to interference.
(ii) PN generator produces periodic sequences that appear to be random.
(iii) PN sequences are generated by an algorithm that uses an initial seed.
(iv) The PN sequence generated is actually not statically random but will pass many test of randomness.
(v) Unless the algorithm and seed are known, the sequence is impractical to predict.

Since, the security level of the watermarking algorithm depends on the strength of its secret key, a gray scale image of size 1×35 is used as a strong key for generating pseudorandom sequences.

Based on the value of the bit of the message vector, the respective two PN sequence pairs are then added/subtracted to/from selective columns of wavelet coefficient. This selection is done by thresholding the coefficient values present in that column. In each selected sub-band, the complete coefficient range is grouped in ten equally spaced bins. The bin having the maximum number of coefficients is chosen for embedding. The embedding procedure of the proposed method is shown in Fig. 6.1.

The column wise DWT coefficients of second level horizontal and vertical sub-bands are taken for embedding. In each column, the coefficients under the threshold criteria are used for embedding and rest of the coefficients remains unchanged. Example embedding process illustrated in Fig. 6.1 shows that values of the coefficients S_2 and S_3 are changed after watermarking as these values lie inside the threshold range while values of coefficient S_1 and S_4 lying outside the threshold criteria remain same. The wavelet coefficients of cover image are divided into k number of *bins* having equal width for desired level. From these k numbers of *bins*, *max_bin*, having maximum number of coefficients is selected. In medical images, DWT coefficients are mostly concentrated toward the origin. Thus, *max_bin* has coefficients concentrated toward origin.

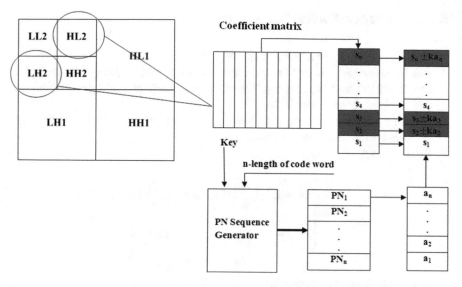

Fig. 6.1 Embedding process of PN sequence in the proposed method

$$\text{Width of each } bin = \frac{\text{maximum coefficient} - \text{minimum coefficient}}{k}$$

b_1 and b_2 are the minimum and maximum values within *max_bin*. In each column, the coefficients under the threshold criteria are used for embedding the data bit as follows:

$$W = V + \alpha \, X \text{ if } b = 0$$

$$W = V - \alpha \, X \text{ if } b = 1$$

where V is DWT coefficient of the cover image, W is the modified DWT coefficient after watermark embedding, α is the gain factor, X is the PN matrix and b is the message bit that has to be embedded. The corresponding column of the DWT coefficient, to which the generated sequence has to be added/subtracted, is decided by the following relation:

$$p = \begin{cases} \text{modulo}\left(d, \dfrac{N}{4}\right) & \text{if modulo}\left(d, \dfrac{N}{4}\right) \neq 0 \\ \dfrac{N}{4}, & \text{else} \end{cases}$$

where p is the column in which sequence has to be added, N/4 is the number of columns in coefficient matrix. Generation of a pair of PN sequences for embedding each bit enhances the security of the watermarking algorithm. In the next subsection process for the embedding of message is discussed.

6.5.1 Message Embedding Algorithm

1. Read the cover image I(M,N) of size M × N.
2. Read the *message* to be hidden and convert it into binary sequences D_d (d=1 to n).
3. Transform the host image using "*Haar*" wavelet transform and get first and second level sub-band coefficients.
4. Generate *n* different PN sequence pairs (PN_h and PN_v) each of $\frac{M}{4} \times 1$ using a secret key to reset the random number generator.
5. for d = 1 to n,

$$
p = \begin{cases} modulo\left(d, \dfrac{N}{4}\right) if\ modulo\left(d, \dfrac{N}{4}\right) \neq 0 \\ \dfrac{N}{4}, \qquad\qquad\qquad\qquad else \end{cases}
$$

Case 1: When message vector bit=0
Hence $1 \leq p \leq (N/4)$, For i=1 to (M/4)

$$
ccH(i,p) = \begin{cases} ccH(i,p) + \alpha \times PN_{h(i,d)}\ if\ b1 < ccH1(i,p) < b2 \\ ccH(i,p) \qquad\qquad\qquad otherwise \end{cases}
$$

$$
ccV(i,p) = \begin{cases} ccV(i,p) + \alpha \times PN\_v(i,d)if\ b1 < ccV1(i,p) < b2 \\ ccV(i,p) \qquad\qquad\qquad otherwise \end{cases}
$$

Case 2: When message vector bit=1
Hence $1 \leq p \leq (N/4)$, For i = 1 to (M/4)

$$
ccH(i,p) = \begin{cases} ccH(i,p) - \alpha \times PN\_h(i,d)if\ b1 < ccH1(i,p) < b2 \\ ccH(i,p) \qquad\qquad\qquad otherwise \end{cases}
$$

$$
ccV(i,p) = \begin{cases} ccV(i,p) - \alpha \times PN\_v(i,d)if\ b1 < ccV1(i,p) < b2 \\ ccV(i,p) \qquad\qquad\qquad otherwise \end{cases}
$$

where α is the gain factor used to specify the strength of the embedded data.

6. Apply inverse "Haar" Wavelet transform to get the final watermarked image $I_w(M, N)$.

6.5.2 Message Extraction Algorithm

The DWT coefficients of watermarked image are divided into k number of bins having equal width for desired level. From this k number of bins, *max_bin*, having maximum number of coefficients is selected. To detect the watermark the same PN sequence vectors used during insertion of watermark are generated by using same state key and determine their correlation with the corresponding selected column's detail sub-bands DWT coefficients. Average of n correlation coefficients corresponding to each PN sequence vector is obtained for both LH and HL sub-bands. Mean of the average correlation values are taken as threshold, T for message extraction. During detection, if the average correlation exceeds T for a particular sequence a "0" is recovered; otherwise a "1". The recovery process then iterates through the entire PN sequence until all the bits of the watermark have been recovered. For extracting the watermark, following steps are applied to the watermarked image:

1. Read the watermarked image $I_w(M, N)$
2. Transform the stego image using "Haar" Wavelet transform and get first and second level sub-band coefficients.
3. Generate one's sequences (*msg*) equal to message vector (from *1* to *n*).
4. Generate n different PN sequence pairs (PN_h1 and PN_v1) each of size $\dfrac{M}{4} \times 1$ using same secret key used in embedding to reset the random number generator.
5. for $d = 1$ to n, Generate PN_h2(d) and PN_v2(d) as

   for $i = 1$ to (M/4)

$$PN\_h2(i,d) = \begin{cases} PN\_h1(i,d) \text{ if } b1 < ccH1(i,p) < b2 \\ 0 \qquad\qquad\qquad\qquad \text{else} \end{cases}$$

$$PN\_v2(i,d) = \begin{cases} PN\_v1(i,d) \text{ if } b1 < ccV1(i,p) < b2 \\ 0 \qquad\qquad\qquad\qquad \text{else} \end{cases}$$

6. Calculate the correlations between the values ccH1 and PN_h2 and store in *corr_H (d)* and ccV1 and PN_v2 *corr_V (d)*.

   corr_H (d) = correlation between PN_h2 (d) and ccH1 (p^{th} column)
   corr_V (d) = correlation between PN_v2 (d) and ccV1 (p^{th} column)

$$p = \begin{cases} \text{modulo}\left(d, \dfrac{N}{4}\right) \text{ if modulo}\left(d, \dfrac{N}{4}\right) \neq 0 \\ \dfrac{N}{4}, \qquad\qquad\qquad\qquad\qquad \text{else} \end{cases}$$

   Hence $1 \leq p \leq \dfrac{N}{4}$

7. Calculate average correlation avg_corr (d) = (corr_H (d)+corr_V(d))/2
8. Calculate the corr(mean) = mean of all the values stored in avg_corr (d).
9. Extract the watermark bit stream, using the relationship given below

for d = 1 to n
if avg_corr (d) > corr (mean)
Msg (d) = 0.

10. Convert the bit sequence to *message watermark* to get the recovered watermark.

6.6   Experimental Results and Performance Analysis

In this section, the performance of combined DWT-SS watermarking algorithm is extensively evaluated for multiple watermarks in the form of image and text. The gray-level MRI image of size 512×512 [15] is taken as the cover image. The health centre logo of "NITK" as image watermark and patient's identity/reference "MRI_1031" as text watermarks. Also, BCH code is applied to the ASCII representation of the text and the encoded text watermark is then embedded. The resulting bits are embedded in two different ways: without ECC and coded by BCH (127, 64) ECC code. The encoded text watermark length for BCH is 127 bits. Strength of watermark is varied by varying the gain factor (α) in the watermarking algorithm. For testing the robustness and quality of the watermarked image of the proposed scheme MATLAB is used. The quality of the watermarked image (as shown in Fig. 6.2) is evaluated by the parameter PSNR and robustness by NC (for image) and BER (text). Figure 6.2 shows the cover MRI image and watermarked images obtained at different gain factors. Extracted watermarks along with the original watermarks are shown in Fig. 6.3. Figure 6.4 shows that larger size watermarks are more clearly identified during extraction.

In the experiments, we are using the gain factor (α) as 1.0 to 5.0 and the value of PSNR, NC and BER are illustrated in Table 6.2, 6.3, 6.4 and 6.5. The performance of the proposed method is better in comparison with the existing [2, 5] method shown in the Table 6.6. In Table 6.2, BCH code performance (determined PSNR and NC values) up to 127 text bits has been evaluated without any noise attack. The maximum PSNR value is 31.92 dB and BER = 0.0472 at α = 1.0 to 5. Figure 6.5 shows the comparison of BER performance as obtained by the proposed method using/without using BCH code. Table 6.3 shows the NC and BER performance of the proposed method against eight different attacks. The highest NC value of 0.7402 has been obtained against the Histogram equalization attack however; the lowest NC is 0.2162 against the Median Filtering attack. The highest BER is obtained as 0.0551 against the Median Filtering attack. However, without BCH code it was 0.0629 for the same attack. It is observed that larger the gain factor, stronger is the robustness and smaller the gain factor, better is the image quality.

Figure 6.6 shows the graphical representation of the BER performance obtained by the proposed method with and without BCH code against different attacks. Table 6.4 shows the effect of watermark size on the PSNR, NC and BER

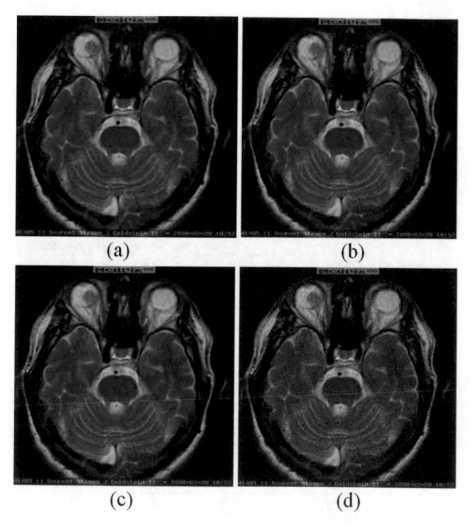

Fig. 6.2 Original and watermarked MRI images (**a**) original image and watermarked images with gain factor; (**b**) 1.0; (**c**) 1.5 and (**d**) 5.0

performance of the proposed watermarking method. It is found that PSNR performance of the watermarked image decreases with the increase in the size of the watermark, but subsequently an improvement in the correlation between original and extracted watermarks is observed. Table 6.5 shows the effect of cover image at $\alpha = 1.5$ on PSNR, NC and BER. The highest NC and BER value were obtained with Ultrasound and MRI image respectively. However, the highest PSNR value (29.82 dB) has been obtained with MRI image. Table 6.6 provides the comparison of PSNR and NC performance obtained by the proposed technique with other reported methods. The maximum NC value with proposed method has been obtained as 0.7544 against 0.659 and 0.3572 obtained by Basant et al. in [2, 5], respectively.

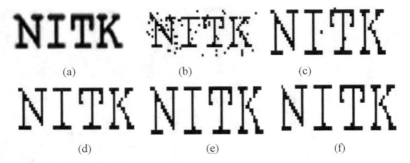

Fig. 6.3 Image watermark (**a**) original and recovered watermark with gain factor α = (**b**) 0.5; (**c**) 1.0; (**d**) 2.5; (**e**) 4.0 and (**f**) 5.0

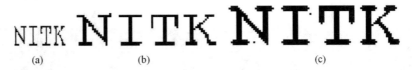

Fig. 6.4 Recovered watermark of different size at gain factor = 5 (**a**) 64 × 20; (**b**) 80 × 25; (**c**) 99 × 31

Table 6.2 Effect of BCH coding on PSNR and BER at different gain factors

Gain factor (α)	Without using BCH coding		Using BCH coding	
	PSNR (dB)	BER (%)	PSNR (dB)	BER (%)
1.0	32.48	0.0629	31.92	0.0472
1.5	29.82	0.0551	28.55	0.0314
2	27.15	0.0472	26.14	0.0314
2.5	25.29	0.0314	24.29	0.0157
3	23.12	0.0078	22.77	0
4	21.94	0.0078	20.40	0
5	19.73	0.0078	18.57	0

The maximum PSNR value obtained with [2, 5] methods are 37.518 dB and 52.04 dB respectively. However, the maximum PSNR value by the proposed method is 37.75 dB. Overall, the proposed method is better than the existing methods [2, 5]. Figure 6.7 shows the graphical representation of the comparison of robustness (determined NC values) offered by the proposed method with that of [2] at different gain factors.

Table 6.3   Effect of BCH coding on NC and BER against different attacks at gain factor (α) = 5

Attacks	Without using BCH coding		Using BCH coding	
	Image watermark (NC value)	Text watermark (BER value in %)	Image watermark (NC value)	Text watermark (BER value in %)
JPEG compression (QF = 10)	0.5306	0.0551	0.5413	0.0314
JPEG compression (QF = 20)	0.7218	0.0393	0.7247	0.0236
JPEG compression (QF = 30)	0.7335	0.0236	0.7335	0
JPEG compression (QF = 50)	0.7364	0.0314	0.7364	0
JPEG compression (QF = 70)	0.7394	0.0236	0.7394	0
JPEG compression (QF = 90)	0.7394	0.0157	0.7394	0
Sharpening mask (threshold = 0.1 and 0.9	0.7394	0.0629 and 0.0472	0.7364	0.0314 and 0
Median filtering [2 2] and [3 3]	0.6736 and 0.2216	0.0629	0.6662 and 0.2162	0.0551 and 0.0472
Scaling factor 2	0.7394	0.0157	0.7364	0
Scaling factor 2.5	0.7394	0.0314	0.7364	0
Scaling factor 5	0.7335	0.0472	0.7335	0.0078
Gaussian LPF (standard deviation = 0.6 and 0.9)	0.7394 and 0.7102	0.0236 and 0.0472	0.7364 and 0.7102	0 and 0.0393
Gaussian noise (mean = 0,Var = 0.01)	0.7335	0.0629	0.7394	0.0157
Gaussian noise (mean = 0,Var = 0.05)	0.6964	0.0551	0.6994	0.0472
Salt & pepper noise (density = 0.02)	0.7391	0.0314	0.7394	0
Salt & pepper noise (density = 0.1)	0.7155	0.0629	0.7072	0.0472
Histogram equalization	0.7394	0	0.7402	0

Table 6.4   Effect of different size of image watermark on PSNR, NC and BER at gain factor (α) = 1.5

Watermark size	Without using BCH coding		
	PSNR (dB)	NC	BER (%)
64 × 20	29.82	0.7394	0.0551
80 × 25	27.03	0.7396	0.0472
99 × 31	23.94	0.9621	0.0472

6.6.1   Performance Evaluation of the Proposed Method for Text Watermarking Using BCH Code

In this subsection, the performance of the above discussed method has been extensively evaluated for text watermark only using BCH code. During the embedding process, the cover image is decomposed up to third level DWT coefficients. For identity authentication purposes, the method uses three different watermarks

Table 6.5 Effect of different cover image on PSNR, NC and BER at gain factor (α) = 1.5

| Cover image | Without using BCH coding | | |
	PSNR (dB)	NC	BER (%)
MRI	29.82	0.7394	0.0551
CT Scan	28.91	0.7384	0.0472
Ultrasound	28.7	0.7395	0.0157

Table 6.6 The comparison results under PSNR and NC value at different gain factors

| Gain factor (α) | Basant et al. [2] | | Basant et al. [5] | | Proposed method | |
	PSNR (dB)	NC	PSNR (dB)	NC	PSNR (dB)	NC
0.5	37.518	0.376	Not reported		37.75	0.6148
1	31.497	0.535	52.04	0.0805	31.92	0.7276
3	21.955	0.657	Not reported		22.77	0.7398
4	19.456	0.659	Not reported		20.4	0.741
5	Not reported		39.02	0.3572	18.57	0.7544

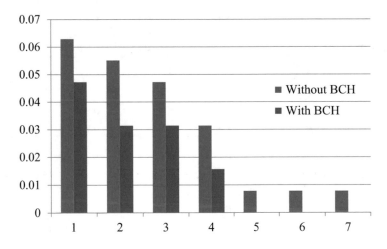

Fig. 6.5 BER performance of the proposed method at different gain factors

representing the text watermark such as personal and medical record of the patient, diagnostic/image codes and doctor code/ signature. According to the importance of robustness requirements, three different text watermarks are embedded into the selected horizontal and vertical sub-band DWT coefficients of the first, second and third level, respectively. Selection of these coefficients for embedding purpose is based on threshold criteria defined above in the chapter. It is found that the proposed scheme correctly extracts the embedded watermarks without error and provides high degree robustness against known attacks while maintaining the imperceptibility of watermarked image.

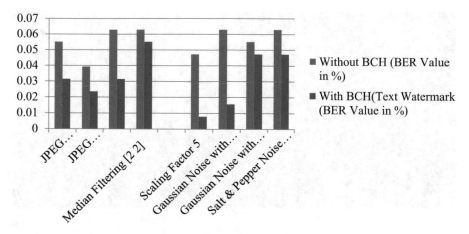

Fig. 6.6 BER performance of the proposed method against different attacks

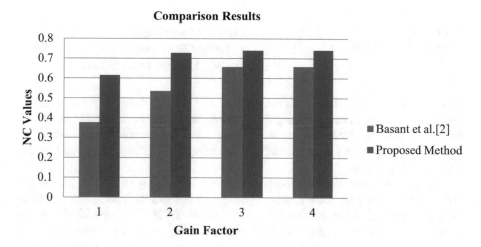

Fig. 6.7 Comparison results under NC values at different gain factors

In this method, the doctor's identification code of eight characters, image/ diagnostic code of eight characters and patient name of eight characters are embedded into third level HL3 and LH3 sub-bands, second level HL2 and LH2 sub-bands and the first level HL1 and LH1 sub-bands respectively. Also, BCH error correcting code is applied to the ASCII representation of the text and the encoded text watermark is then embedded into the cover medical images. The resulting bits are embedded in two different ways: without ECC and coded by BCH (127, 64) code. Performance of the proposed method has been extensively evaluated against known attacks and results are compared with other technique [10]. The proposed method gives superior robustness performance without significant degradation of the image quality of the watermarked image. The encoded text watermark length for BCH is

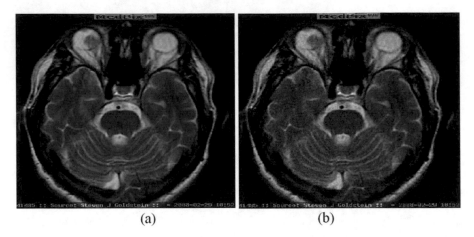

(a)   (b)

Fig. 6.8 (**a**) Cover image (**b**) Watermarked image at gain factor (α) = 15

Fig. 6.9 Extracted text
watermark at gain factor
(α) = 15

Doctor's identification code: BXBPS495
Image/ Diagnostic code: NITK_196
Patient' name: AmitKrS

381 bits. The strength of the watermark is tested by varying the gain factor (α) in the watermarking algorithm. Imperceptibility performance of the scheme is evaluated by calculating the PSNR between cover image and watermarked image where as robustness performance is measured by calculating BER between original and the extracted watermark.

Fig. 6.8 shows original MRI image and watermarked image at α = 15. Figure 6.9 shows the extracted watermark image at α = 15. PSNR and BER performance of the proposed watermarking scheme with and without BCH coder are illustrated in Table 6.7. Referring this table it is observed that the highest PSNR obtained without and with BCH coder are 43.96 dB and 40.48 dB respectively (at α = 5) whereas BER obtained without and with BCH coder are 0.0236 and 0.0183 respectively. It is also observed that the watermarking scheme with BCH coder achieves desired '0' BER at gain factor of 15 but its PSNR performance is slightly compromised i.e. 29.46 dB as compared to 34.95 dB achieved without coder.

In Table 6.8, robustness performance of the proposed algorithm with and without BCH coder has been tested at α = 10 against different attacks. With BCH coder, BER value = 0 is obtained against JPEG compression (Quality Factor (QF) = 90) whereas without BCH code it comes out to be 0.0052. It is also observed from the table that the implementation of BCH coder improves the BER performance for sharpening mask noise attack with threshold = 1. Table 6.9 shows PSNR and BER performance of the proposed algorithm for different imaging modalities at varying gain factor. It is observed that Ultrasound image gives maximum PSNR = 41.30 dB at gain factor of 5 whereas minimum BER value = '0' is obtained with MRI image at gain factor of 11. Table 6.10 provides the performance (determined PSNR and

Table 6.7 PSNR and BER performance of the proposed method with and without BCH code

Gain factors (α)	Without using BCH coding		Using BCH coding	
	PSNR (dB)	BER value (%)	PSNR	BER value (%)
5	43.96	0.0236	40.48	0.0183
10	38.43	0.0078	31.31	0.0052
15	34.95	0.0052	29.46	0
20	32.66	0	29.01	0

Table 6.8 BER performance of proposed method with and without BCH code against different attacks at gain factor (α) = 10

Attacks	Without using BCH coding	Using BCH coding
	BER value (%)	BER value (%)
JPEG compression (QF = 90)	0.0052	0
JPEG compression (QF = 50)	0.0183	0.0131
JPEG compression (QF = 30)	0.0157	0.0183
JPEG compression (QF = 15)	0.0367	0.0314
JPEG compression (QF = 5)	0.0629	0.0603
Sharpening mask (threshold = 1.0)	0.0052	0
Median filtering [2 2] and [3 3]	0.0236 and 0.0446	0.0183 and 0.0367
Gaussian LPF (standard deviation = 0.5)	0.0157	0.0131
Gaussian noise (mean = 0,Var = 0.01)	0.0288	0.0209
Gaussian noise (mean = 0,Var = 0.1)	0.0367	0.0314
Salt & pepper noise (density = 0.001)	0	0
Salt & pepper noise (density = 0.05)	0.0314	0.0262
Motion Blur (Len = 9, Theta = 0)	0.0314	0.0288

BER values) comparison with the existing methods. The maximum BER value with proposed method has been obtained as zero against 1.5306 obtained by Kumar et al. in [10] method. The maximum PSNR value is obtained with this method is 45.51 dB. However, the maximum PSNR value is obtained by the proposed method is 49.12 dB. The existing method [10] can embed only 196 bits only whereas 381 bits can be embedded by the proposed method. Overall, the proposed method is better than the existing method in terms of image quality of the watermarked image, robustness of the extracted watermark and embedding capacity also.

From the above extensive discussion, we have observed some important remarks:

As shown in Table 6.3, the highest value of NC = 0.7402 is obtained for Histogram equalization attack whereas its lowest value of 0.2162 is achieved for median filtering attack. The lowest BER value 0 is obtained for JPEG compression (QF = 30, 50, 70, 90), Sharpening mask (threshold = 0.9), Scaling factor (2 and 2.5), Gaussian LPF (standard deviation = 0.6), Salt and pepper noise (density = 0.02) and Histogram equalization attacks, however, higher value of BER = 0.0551 is observed for median filtering attack. The higher robustness as indicated by NC value = 0.7544 is achieved

Table 6.9 Effect of cover images on PSNR and BER performance at different gain factors

Cover image	Gain factor (α) = 5		Gain factor (α) = 11		Gain factor (α) = 15	
	PSNR (dB)	BER value (%)	PSNR (dB)	BER value (%)	PSNR (dB)	BER value (%)
MRI	40.47	0.0209	33.83	0	31.3	0
CT Scan	41.15	0.0183	34.49	0.0131	31.79	0
Ultrasound	41.3	0.0157	34.65	0	31.95	0

Table 6.10 The comparison results under PSNR and BER value

Gain factor	Kumar et al. [10]		Proposed method	
	PSNR (dB)	BER value (%)	PSNR (dB)	BER value (%)
3	45.51	1.5306	49.12	0
5	41.07	0	45.76	0
10	35.05	0	39.01	0
15	31.53	0	35.35	0

in our proposed method as compared to other reported techniques [2, 5]. Referring Table 6.6 it is seen that maximum value of NC = 0.7544 is achieved at gain factor 'α' = 5 as compared to its corresponding maximum NC values of '0.6590' and '0.3572' in [2, 5] respectively. Further, it is also evident from Table 6.6 that the proposed method offers up to 63.51% superior performance in terms of robustness over reported techniques [2, 5]. The performance of the proposed watermarking method has been extensively evaluated only for text watermark at multilevel DWT sub-bands. This is carried out by applying BCH code on the EPR data as text watermark before embedding into the cover. The BER of the text watermark has been evaluated against different known attacks as in Table 6.8. The BER = 0 is obtained for JPEG compression (QF = 90), sharpening mask (threshold = 1.0) and Salt and pepper noise (density = 0.001), however, higher value of BER = 0.0603 is obtained for JPEG compression attacks (QF = 5). The PSNR and BER performance of the proposed method is also compared with [10] as shown in Table 6.10 from which it is evident that the proposed method offers up to 7.93% enhancement in visual quality of the watermarked image and 1.53% reduction in BER over [10].

6.6.2 Performance Evaluation of Proposed Method Using Multilevel Encrypted Text Watermarking

In order to enhance the security of the text watermark, reduce save the massage encryption/decryption time and address the health data management issues, the encrypted text watermark is embedding into the appropriated DWT sub-bands. In this subsection, simultaneous embedding of three watermarks (i.e. doctor code,

Table 6.11 Allocation of watermarks according to robustness and capacity criteria at different sub-band

DWT sub-band	Capacity (embeddable coefficients)	Embedded watermark	
		EPR data	Robustness requirements
LH3	4096	Identification code of the doctor and Patient's diagnostic/image codes	Very high
HL3	4096	Identification code of the doctor and Patient's diagnostic/image codes	Very high
LH2	16384	Patient's medical and personal records	High
HL2	16384	Patient's medical records	High

image reference code and patient record) using multilevel watermarking of cover medical image has been proposed to address the issues of medical data confidentiality, data security, data compaction, unauthorized access and temper proofing. The suggested method uses wavelet based spread-spectrum watermarking where the encrypted text watermarks are embedded at multiple levels of the DWT sub-bands of the cover image. The performance of the developed scheme was evaluated and analyzed against known attacks by varying watermark size and the gain factor. It is found that the proposed multilevel watermarking method enhances the security of the patient data. The advantage of the work is summarized as follows:

(i) *Improved capacity*: The method proposed by Basant et al. [10] and Singh et al. [13] has been embedded 196 and 381 bits respectively. However, in our proposed method we can embed 728 bits (116 characters) with the acceptable performance in terms of robustness and imperceptibility.

(ii) *Enhanced security of the text watermark*: security of the medical text watermark may be enhanced by using simple encryption method to save execution time. For tele-diagnosis, the encryption and decryption speed has become an important factor if the situation demands.

(iii) *Reduced bandwidth requirements*: The EPR data in the form of three different text watermarks are embedding in the same medical cover image which reduce the bandwidth requirements as essential importance in medical applications

(iv) *Health data management*: Further, the proposed method addressing the medical data management issues data security, data compaction, unauthorized access and temper proofing, having different characteristics and requirements. This has been achieved by allocation of watermarks according to robustness and capacity requirements at different DWT sub-band of the cover image. The allocation of the watermarks is presented in Table 6.11 [16].

In this method, the personal and medical record of the patient is embedded into selected sub-bands of the second level. However, identification code of the doctor and patient's diagnostic/image codes of the patient are embedded into selected sub-bands of the third level. The doctor identification and image reference codes are embedded into third level HL3 and LH3 sub-bands, while the patient record is embedded into HL2 and LH2 sub-bands of second level DWT sub-band. Also, encryption is applied to the ASCII representation of the text watermark and the encrypted text watermark is then embedded. Thus, the method enhances security of the text watermark. The encryption method used in the present work is simple to reduce the execution time during encryption and decryption. The EPR data is encrypted and decrypted using the equations 1 and 2, respectively as given in section "Encryption and decryption process for text watermark" of chapter "Robust and Imperceptible Hybrid Watermarking Techniques for Medical Images".

The performance of the proposed watermarking method was tested for encrypted text medical watermark considering gray–level medical images of size 512×512 [15] as cover image. Two different text watermarks doctor identification code of ten characters and radiological image reference code of five characters are embedded into third level HL3 and LH3 sub-bands, while the patient record of varying size is embedded into HL2 and LH2 sub-bands of second level DWT as the third watermark. Encryption is applied to the ASCII representation of these text watermarks and the encrypted text watermarks are then embedded providing the extra level of security during embedding process. The strength of watermark is varied by varying the gain factor (α) in the watermarking algorithm. Figure 6.10 shows the cover CT Scan image and watermarked images obtained at different gain factors. Figure 6.11 shows the EPR data using as text watermarks. In the experiment, values of PSNR and BER are illustrated in Tables 6.12, 6.13, and 6.14 for varying gain factors (α) in the range of 5.0 to 15.0.

Table 6.12 shows the effect of gain factor on the performance (determined PSNR and BER values) of the proposed method for different sizes of watermark. With the encryption, maximum PSNR value is 40.02 dB and BER = 0.1538 against maximum size of watermark at $\alpha = 5$. However, PSNR value is 31.05 dB and BER = 0 at $\alpha = 15$.

Table 6.13 shows the effect of encryption on BER performance as obtained by the proposed multilevel watermarking method against ten different attacks. The highest BER value of 0.3846 is obtained against JPEG compression attack with quality factor (QF) = 10 with encryption which is slightly better than the BER performance without encryption (BER = 0.4326). Further, from Table 6.3 it is evident that the proposed technique reduces BER up to 0.124% while providing extra level of security of the text watermark using encryption compared to the method without using the encryption of text watermark.

Table 6.14 shows the effect of cover medical images on PSNR and BER performance as obtained by the proposed method at gain factor (α) = 15. It is observed that the highest PSNR and BER were obtained with MRI image, which is also shown in Figs. 6.12 and 6.13, respectively. Figure 6.14 shows BER performance of the proposed multilevel watermarking method against known attacks at gain factor (α) = 15.

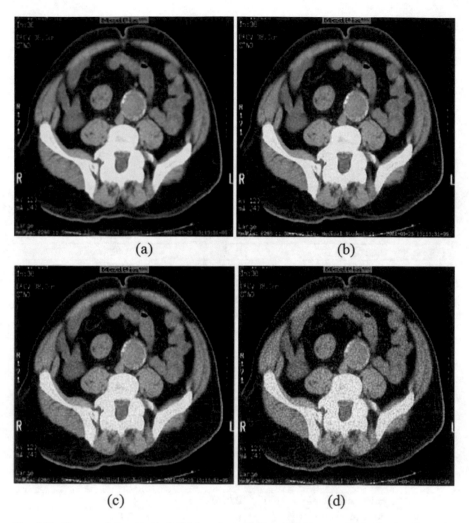

Fig. 6.10 Cover and watermarked CT Scan images (**a**) original image and watermarked images with gain factor; (**b**) 5; (**c**) 15 and (**d**) 40

Doctor's and Image code: BXBPS4951D_NIT01
Patient's Record:
OPD_051_NITKurukshetra_Stroke_amennea_BPositive_AmitSingh_20-05-
80_DrBasantKumar_2017

Fig. 6.11 EPR data as text watermark

Table 6.12 Effect of gain factor on PSNR and BER for different sizes of watermark

Gain factor (α)	With encryption				Without encryption			
	104 characters		60 characters		104 characters		60 characters	
	PSNR (dB)	BER (%)	PSNR (dB)	BER (%)	PSNR (dB)	BER (%)	PSNR (dB)	BER (%)
5	40.02	0.1538	42.49	0.0961	40.06	0.1923	42.53	0.1250
10	34.24	0.0576	36.71	0.0288	34.27	0.0769	36.8	0.0480
15	31.05	0	33.29	0	31.08	0.0192	33.32	0.0096

Table 6.13 Effect of encryption on BER for different attacks at gain factor (α) = 15

Attack	With encryption BER (%) for 104 characters	Without encryption BER (%) for 104 characters
JPEG compression (QF = 10)	0.3846	0.4326
JPEG compression (QF = 50)	0.0096	0.0288
JPEG compression (QF = 90)	0	0.0192
Sharpening mask (threshold = 0.2 and 0.1)	0.0192 and 0	0.0288
Median filtering [3 3] and [2 2]	0.0480 and 0	0.0769 and 0.0288
Scaling factor 2.5,1.5 and 0.5	0.0769, 0.0576 and 0	0.1057, 0.0673 and 0.0288
Motion Blur (len = 2 and theta = 9)	0.0192	0.0192
Motion Blur (len = 1 and theta = 9)	0	0.0192
Disk (radius = 1)	0.0288	0.0480
Disk (radius = 0.5)	0	0.0192
Gaussian LPF (standard deviation = 0.2,0.5 and 0.9)	0, 0.0096 and 0.0673	0.0192, 0.0192 and 0.0865
Gaussian noise (mean = 0,Var = 0.05)	0.0769	0.1057
Gaussian noise (mean = 0,Var = 0.01)	0.0288	0.0480
Gaussian noise (mean = 0,Var = 0.005)	0	0.0192
Salt & pepper noise with (density = 0.05)	0.0961	0.1153
Salt & pepper noise (density = 0.01)	0.0288	0.0384
Salt & pepper Noise (density = 0.005)	0	0.0192
Histogram equalization	0.0961	0.1250

Table 6.14 PSNR and BER performance using different cover images at gain factor (α) = 15

Cover image	With encryption	
	PSNR (dB)	BER (%)
CT Scan	31.03	0
Ultrasound	30.37	0
MRI	31.23	0.0480

Fig. 6.12 PSNR
performance of proposed
method using different
cover images

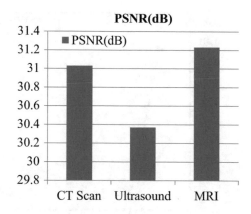

Fig. 6.13 BER
performance of the
proposed method using
different cover images

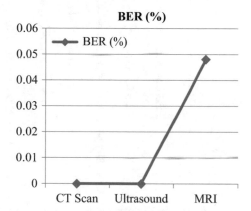

6.6.3   *Performance Evaluation of the Proposed Method for Image and Text Watermarking Using Encryption and BCH Code Simultaneously*

The performance of the method is also tested for multiple watermarks using encryption and BCH code simultaneously. For the extensive analysis of the proposed work, we have tested the method with some minor changes as follows:

1) The methods discussed in Sects. 6.1 and 6.2 using threshold criteria for the embedding purpose. However, the watermark bits are embedding here without using the threshold criteria.
2) The method using the same algorithm for image watermark, as disused in Sect. 6.5. However, the text watermark embedding and extraction process is different, as discussed detail in [17].

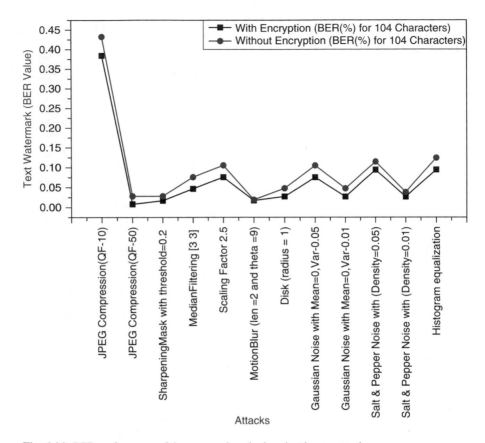

Fig. 6.14 BER performance of the proposed method against known attacks

In this context, the method adopts to extend two existing single watermarking techniques [5, 17] to achieve several goals in medical image watermarking like security, high capacity and robustness. Figure 6.15 show the embedding process of the proposed technique. The proposed dual watermarking algorithm embeds *health centre's logo as image watermark* using spread spectrum watermarking technique and embedding of sensitive *patient's information* as text watermark (up to 150 Characters) into the high frequency component (HH2 Sub-band) of the DWT cover image is considered.

Further, the proposed dual watermarking method is embedding two different watermarks in cover medical image simultaneously, which has fewer constraints than the other two dual watermarks methods [18–20]. The main contribution of the work is summarized as follow:

(i) *Dual watermarking and improved capacity*: The method reported in [6, 21–29] has embedded only one watermark. The proposed technique is embedding multiple watermarks simultaneously in non-interfering way [20] to enhance the security and capacity of the hidden watermark and reduce the bandwidth

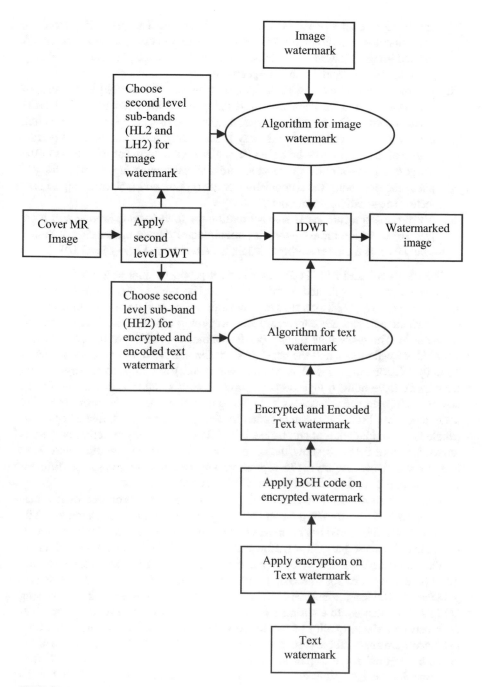

Fig. 6.15 Proposed dual watermark embedding method

and storage requirements for medical applications. The proposed technique can embeds up to 150 characters with acceptable visual quality of the watermarked image. However, the methods reported in [10, 13, 16] can embed only 196 bits, 381 bits and 728 bits respectively.

(ii) *Improved performance*: In Table 6.18, robustness and security performance of text watermark have been improved using encryption technique and BCH channel coding. Further, the encryption technique [14] along with BCH coding based method is compared with only BCH coding based method and performance of the proposed scheme has been observed in terms of robustness of the image and text watermark against different signal processing attacks. The proposed method using the combination of encryption and watermarking to protecting the sensitive patient data.

(iii) The proposed technique is also addressing the *health data management issue* [14, 16] in which more important patient/doctor data is embedding at higher level DWT and the less important data is embedding at lower level DWT.

The PSNR NC and BER Performance of the proposed dual watermarking algorithm is extensively evaluated for medical data. The 8-bit grey scale MR image of size 512×512 [15], health centre's logo of different sizes and patient's information of 150 characters and are considered as cover image, image and text watermark respectively. The perceptual quality (as determined by PSNR) of the cover image with hidden watermark and the robustness of the extracted watermarks (as determine by NC for image and BER for text watermark) is evaluated at varying gain factors. We have noticed that the perceptual quality is better at lower gain factor, however, stronger the robustness at higher gain values. In BCH error correcting code, redundant bit information is added in binary sequence such that error is distributed over redundant bits and hence, the BER value in the extraction process is reduced. Figure 6.16a, b show the cover MR and watermark health centre logo image respectively. Figure 6.17a–c presents the watermarked images at different gain factors. Figure 6.18 show the patient data as text watermark.

Table 6.15 shows the PSNR and NC performance of the proposed dual watermarking method at different gain factors using varying number of characters. The highest PSNR (38.63 dB) has been obtained for the maximum size of the text watermark (151 characters) at gain = 1. However, highest NC (0.8673) has been obtained for the same size of the text watermark at gain = 7. Referring this table, it is observed that PSNR decreases for increasing number of characters embedded and chosen gain factors. However, robustness (NC values) of the image watermark is increasing at higher gain factors. In addition, the value of gain factor = 5 provides a good balance between visual quality of the watermarked image and the robustness of the extracted watermark. Table 6.16 shows the PSNR, NC and BER performance of the proposed method for different sizes of the image watermark at gain = 5. It is observed that the NC values have been found ranges from 0.5794 to 0.8026 for different size of image watermark. However, BER for recovered text watermark (size = 145 characters = 1015 bits) is '0' for all cases using BCH error correcting code, indicating a perfect recovery of the text watermark. Table 6.17 presents the PSNR,

Fig. 6.16 (a) Cover MR and (b) watermark logo image

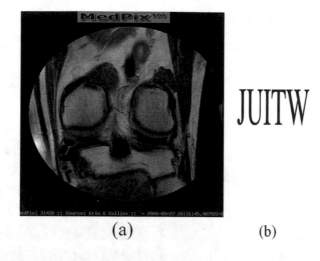

(a)   (b)

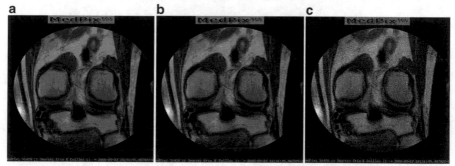

Fig. 6.17 Watermarked MR image at (a) Gain = 1 (b) Gain = 5 and (b) Gain = 15

NC and BER performance of the proposed method for different cover images such as MRI, Brain CT Scan, Ultrasound, Barbara and Lena images at gain factor = 5. In this table, the PSNR values are above than 30.00 dB for all the considered cover images. The highest PSNR were obtained with Lena image (PSNR = 37.04dB). The range of NC values from 0.7254 to 0.8657. The highest NC value were obtained for MRI image (NC = 0.8657). However, the lowest NC value were obtained for CT Scan image (NC = 0.7254). Referring this table, it is observed that all the BER values have been found '0' except the Ultrasound image which is greater than '0'.

Table 6.18 shows the NC and BER performance of the proposed dual watermarking method against known attacks at gain factor = 3 using text bits = 140. Without using the encryption, the highest NC value (0.9615) has been obtained for Gaussian LPF and sharpening mask and the lowest NC value of 0.3498 is obtained against salt and pepper attacks. The highest BER (12.85%) has been found against median filtering attack, whereas lowest BER (0%) is found against Gaussian low pass filtering, sharpening mask, JPEG compression, histogram equalization and cropping. Referring this table, it is observed that all the NC values (with encryption) is greater

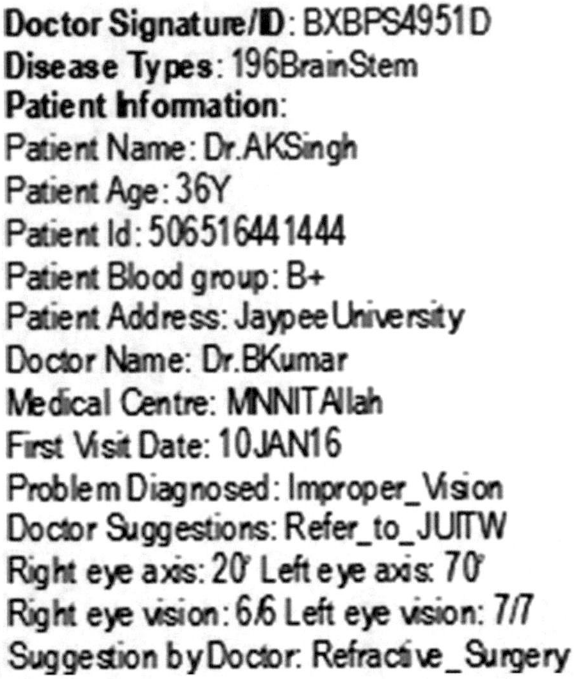

Fig. 6.18 Patient
information as text
watermark

Doctor Signature/ID: BXBPS4951D
Disease Types: 196BrainStem
Patient Information:
Patient Name: Dr.AKSingh
Patient Age: 36Y
Patient Id: 506516441444
Patient Blood group: B+
Patient Address: Jaypee University
Doctor Name: Dr.BKumar
Medical Centre: MNNITAllah
First Visit Date: 10JAN16
Problem Diagnosed: Improper_Vision
Doctor Suggestions: Refer_to_JUITW
Right eye axis: 20° Left eye axis: 70°
Right eye vision: 6/6 Left eye vision: 7/7
Suggestion by Doctor: Refractive_Surgery

than the NC values as obtained without using the encryption method except for
Gaussian LPF and sharpening mask. Table 6.19 presents the NC and BER performance of the proposed dual watermarking method against known attacks at gain
factor = 5 using text bits = 1015. It is observed that all the NC values (with encryption) are greater than 0.7 except for Gaussian Noise (Mean = 0, Var-0.01), Salt &
Pepper Noise (with density = 0.05), JPEG Compression (QF-10), Median Filtering
(3 x 3). It is also observed that the BER performance is highly dependent on the
noise variations. The results indicate that the proposed dual watermarking method
is robust against various signal processing attacks. In addition, the performance of
the proposed method highly depends on size of the watermarks, gain factor and
noise variations.

6.7 Summary

In this chapter, the authors presents spread-spectrum based methods for secure multiple watermarking of medical images in wavelet domain which simultaneously
embeds text and image both or text watermarks only into a cover medical image.
The use of spread-spectrum technique secures the image watermark whereas
improvement in robustness of the text watermark has been achieved using BCH
code before embedding. Experimental results were obtained by varying watermark

Table 6.15 PSNR, NC and BER Performance of the proposed method at different gain factors

Gain factor	PSNR (dB)				NC					BER			
	20 char	40 char	123 char	151	20 char	40 char	123 char	151 char		20 char	40 char	123 char	151 char
1	39.51	39.10	38.63	38.63	0.3776	0.3814	0.3902	0.3886		0	0	0	0.0066
3	36.01	35.82	35.59	35.59	0.7118	0.7131	0.7118	0.7093		0	0	0	0.0066
5	32.77	32.68	32.57	32.57	0.8181	0.8181	0.8174	0.8159		0	0	0	0.0132
7	30.25	30.20	30.14	30.14	0.8682	0.8690	0.8665	0.8673		0	0	0	0.0132

Table 6.16 PSNR, NC and BER Performance of the proposed method at different size of the image watermark

Size of image watermark	PSNR (dB)	NC	BER (%)
50 × 12	36.33	0.6257	0
85 × 19	33.69	0.8026	0
89 × 19	33.57	0.8009	0
100 × 25	32.28	0.7204	0
100 × 40	30.6	0.5794	0

Table 6.17 PSNR, NC and BER Performance of the proposed method for different cover image

Cover image	PSNR (dB)	NC	BER (%)
Medimix	35.93	0.81.59	0
MRI	33.15	0.8657	0
CT Scan	31.87	0.7254	0
Ultra sound	32.97	0.7991	0.1310
Lena	37.04	0.8362	0
Barbara	30.19	0.7802	0

Table 6.18 NC and BER performance of the proposed method against different attacks

Attacks	Using BCH and without using encryption		With BCH and encryption	
	NC	BER	NC	BER (%)
Gaussian noise (M = 0,V = 0.01)	0.3568	5	0.5091	0.1
Salt & pepper noise (D = 5%)	0.3498	8.5714	0.4416	0.2
Gaussian LPF (STD = 0.6)	0.9615	0	0.6435	0
Gaussian LPF (std = 0.5)			0.6729	0
Scaling (F = 6)	0.6758	7.1429	0.6703	0.15
Sharpening mask (threshold = 0.8 and 0.1)	0.9615	0	0.7922 and 0.8062	0
JPEG compression (QF-90)	0.6831	0	0.6868	0
JPEG compression (QF-70)	0.6397	0	0.6424	0
JPEG compression (QF-50)	0.6059	0	0.6091	0
Median filtering [2 2]	0.5631	12.85	0.5541	0
Histogram equalization	0.7838	0	0.7859	0

size, gain factor and medical cover image modalities. The performance of the developed technique was tested against the known attacks. The method is also compared with other reported techniques and has been found to be giving superior performance for robustness with acceptable perceptual quality of the watermarked image suggested by other reported techniques. The proposed method offers up to 63.51% superior performance in terms of robustness over other reported techniques.

Table 6.19 NC and BER performance of the proposed method for different attacks

Attacks	Proposed technique	
	NC	BER
Gaussian noise (M = 0,V = 0.0001)	0.8094	0.034
Gaussian noise (M = 0,V = 0.001)	0.7800	0.282
Gaussian noise (M = 0,V = 0.01)	0.6598	0.841
Salt & pepper noise (D = 0.001)	0.8124	0
Salt & pepper noise (D = 0.005)	0.7788	0.0413
Salt & pepper noise (D = 0.05)	0.5904	0.724
Gaussian LPF (std = 0.05)	0.8151	0
Gaussian LPF (std = 0.1)	0.8159	0
Gaussian LPF (std = 0.5)	0.7894	0.0068
Scaling (F = 2)	0.7911	0.2551
Sharpening mask (threshold = 0.8 and 0.1)	0.8879 and 0.8706	0.0827 and 0.0620
JPEG compression (QF-90)	0.802	0
JPEG compression (QF-50)	0.7559	0.4068
JPEG compression (QF-10)	0.4656	0.9793
Median filtering [2 2] and [3 3]	0.7047 and 0.6837	0.7655 and 0.6620
Histogram equalization	0.8596	0.0413

Further, the performance of the proposed watermarking method has been extensively evaluated only for text watermark at multilevel DWT sub-bands by applying
BCH code on the watermark considered as EPR data before embedding into the
cover has been investigated. The performance of the developed technique was tested
against the known attacks. The PSNR and BER performance of the proposed method
is also compared with other reported technique. It is evident that the proposed
method offers up to 7.93% enhancement in visual quality of the watermarked image
and 1.53% reduction in BER over the reported techniques. Moreover, the method is
also addressing the health data management issue where the encrypted text watermarks are embedded at multiple levels of the DWT sub-bands of the cover image.
From the above discussion, we have observed that method reduces BER up to
0.124% while providing extra level of security of the text watermark using encryption method. Moreover, the performance of the method is also tested for multiple
watermarks using encryption and BCH code simultaneously.

The proposed techniques is providing a potential solution to existing problem of
secure medical data transmission over open and bandwidth constrained network. It
also deals the problem of patient identity theft, which is a growing and dangerous
concern in this area. For improvement in error correction capability of extracted text
watermark bits, length of the error correction code may be suitably increased.
Correlation and security of the method can be improved further by using other
extended PN sequences such as random sequence, maximal length sequence, gold
sequence and Kasami sequence.

References

1. O. Vikas, Multilingualism for cultural diversity and universal access in cyberspace: an Asian perspective, UNESCO, May 2005
2. B. Kumar, H.V. Singh, S.P. Singh, A. Mohan, Secure spread-spectrum watermarking for telemedicine applications. J. Inf. Security **2**(2), 91–98 (2011)
3. G. Coatrieux, H. Maitre, B. Sankur, Y. Rolland, R. Collorec, Relevance of watermarking in medical imaging, in Proceeding of the Information Technology Applications in Biomedicine, pp. 250–255, 2000
4. C. Pujara, A. Bhardwaj, V.M. Gadre, Secured watermarking fractional wavelet domains. IETE J. Res. **53**(6), 573–580 (2007)
5. B. Kumar, A. Anand, S.P. Singh, A. Mohan, High capacity spread-spectrum watermarking for telemedicine applications. World Acad. Sci. Eng. Technol. **5**, 58–62 (2011)
6. I.J. Cox, J. Kilian, F.T. Leighton, T. Shamoon, Secure spread spectrum watermarking for multimedia. IEEE Trans. Image Process. **6**(12), 1673–1687 (1997)
7. H.S. Malvar, D.A.F. Florencio, Improved spread spectrum: a new modilation technique for robust watermarking. IEEE Trans. Signal Process. **51**(4), 898–905 (2003)
8. L. Perez-Freire, F. Perez-Gonzalez, Spread-spectrum watermarking security. IEEE Trans. Inf. Forensics Security **4**(1), 2–24 (2009)
9. G. Xuan, C. Yang, Y. Zheng, Y.Q. Shi, Z. Ni, Reversible data hiding based on wavelet spread spectrum, in IEEE International Workshop on Multimedia Signal Processing, Siena, Italy, pp. 211–214, 2004
10. B. Kumar, S.B. Kumar, D.S. Chauhan, Wavelet based imperceptible medical image watermarking using spread-spectrum, in Proceeding of 37th International Conference on Telecommunications and Signal Processing, Berlin, Germany, pp. 660–664, 2014
11. J. Domingo-Ferrer, F. Sebé, Invertible spread-spectrum watermarking for image authentication and multilevel access to precision-critical watermarked images, in Proceedings of the International Conference on Information Technology: Coding and Computing, pp. 1–6, 2002
12. T.S. Das, V.H. Mankar, S.K. Sarkar, Spread spectrum based robust image watermark authentication, in International Conference, Madurai, India, pp. 673–676, 2007
13. A.K. Singh, B. Kumar, M. Dave, A. Mohan, Robust and imperceptible spread-spectrum watermarking for telemedicine applications. Proc. Natl. Acad. Sci., India, Sect. A: Phys. Sci. (2015). doi:10.1007/s40010-014-0197-6
14. A.K. Singh, M. Dave, A. Mohan, Multilevel encrypted text watermarking on medical images using spread-spectrum in DWT domain. Wirel. Pers. Commun. **83**(3), 2133–2150 (2015)
15. MedPix TM Medical Image Database available at http://rad.usuhs.mil/medpix/medpix.html
16. A. Giakoumaki, S. Pavlopoulos, D. Koutsouris, Secure and efficient health data management through multiple watermarking on medical images. Med. Biol. Eng. Comput. **44**, 619–631 (2006)
17. N. Terzija, M. Repges, K. Luck, W. Geisselhardt, Digital image watermarking using DWT: performance comparison on error correcting codes, in Visualization, Imaging, and Image Processing Proceeding (364), 2002
18. K. Wu, W. Yan, J. Du, A robust dual digital-image watermarking technique, in International Conference on Computational Intelligence and Security Workshop, pp. 668–671, 2007
19. C. Chemak, M.S. Bouhlel, J.C. Lapayre, A new scheme of robust image watermarking: the double watermarking algorithm, in Proceedings of the 2007 Summer Computer Simulation Conference, SCSC 2007, San Diego, CA, USA, pp. 1201–1208, 2007
20. H. Shen, B. Chen, From single watermark to dual watermark: a new approach for image watermarking. Comput. Electr. Eng. **38**, 1310–1324 (2012)
21. A. Singh, A. Tayal, Choice of wavelet from wavelet families for DWT–DCT–SVD image watermarking. Int. J. Comput. Appl. **48**(17), 9–14 (2012)

22. M.I. Khan, M.M. Rahman, M.I.H. Sarker, Digital watermarking for image authentication based on combined DCT, DWT, and SVD transformation. Int. J. Comput. Sci. **10**(5), 223–230 (2013)
23. A. Srivastava, P. Saxena, DWT-DCT-SVD based semi blind image watermarking using middle frequency band. IOSR J. Computer Eng. **12**(2), 63–66 (2013)
24. N.J. Harish, B.B.S. Kumar, A. Kusagur, Hybrid robust watermarking techniques based on DWT, DCT, and SVD. Int. J. Adv. Electr. Electron. Eng. **2**(5), 137–143 (2013)
25. B.L. Gunjal, R.R. Manthalkar, An overview of transform domain robust digital image watermarking algorithms. J. Emerg. Trends Computer Inf. Sci. **2**(1), 13–16 (2011)
26. F. Chen, H. He, Y. Huo, H. Wang, Self-recovery fragile watermarking scheme with variable watermark payload, Proceedings of the 10th International Conference on Digital-Forensics and Watermarking, Atlantic City, NY, pp. 142–155, 2011
27. N.H. Divecha, N.N. Jani, Image watermarking algorithm using DCT, DWT and SVD, in *Proceedings on National Conference on Innovative Paradigms in Engineering and Technology*, vol. 10, 2012, pp. 13–16
28. K.A. Navas, A.M. Cheriyan, M. Lekshmi, S.A. Tampy, M. Sasikumar, DWT–DCT–SVD based watermarking, in Proceedings of the 3rd International Conference on Communication Systems Software and Middleware and Workshop, Bangalore, pp. 271–274, 2008
29. B. Wang, J. Ding, Q. Wen, X. Liao, C. Liu, An image watermarking algorithm based on DWT DCT and SVD, in IEEE International Conference on Network Infrastructure and Digital Content, Beijing, pp. 1034–1038, 2009

Chapter 7
Robust and Secure Multiple Watermarking Technique for Application in Tele-Ophthalmology

Amit Kumar Singh, Basant Kumar, Ghanshyam Singh, and Anand Mohan

7.1 Introduction

Recently, rapid advances in information and communication technology (ICT) have facilitated newer telemedicine services by supporting open channel communications for cost effective and speedy transmission of electronic patient record (EPR) to remote hospitals/medical consultation centers [1, 2]. However, such type of exchange of EPR for diagnostic applications faces the challenging risk of authenticity, confidentiality, and ownership identity due to attempts of malicious attacks or hacking of EPR either to alter/modify the original patient record or even to prevent its transfer to intended recipients. The authenticity of EPR and related medical images are generally ensured in telemedicine applications by embedding some kind of watermark(s). Therefore, authentication and preservation of originality of a patient's record requires robust and secure embedding of the watermark(s) against attempts of unauthorized

A.K. Singh (✉)
Department of Computer Science & Engineering, Jaypee University of Information
Technology, Waknaghat, Solan, India
e-mail: amit_245singh@yahoo.com

B. Kumar
Department of Electronics and Communication Engineering, Motilal Nehru National
Institute of Technology, Allahabad, India
e-mail: singhbasant@yahoo.com

G. Singh
Department of Electronics and Communication Engineering, Jaypee University
of Information Technology, Waknaghat, Solan, India
e-mail: drghanshyam.singh@yahoo.com

A. Mohan
Department of Electronics Engineering, Indian Institute of Technology (BHU),
Varanasi, India
e-mail: profanandmohan@gmail.com

© Springer International Publishing AG 2017
A.K. Singh et al. (eds.), *Medical Image Watermarking*, Multimedia Systems
and Applications, DOI 10.1007/978-3-319-57699-2_7

access or modification of medical data transmitted over open channels. In view of the above and considering wide applications of tele-ophthalmology as well as its related security concerns, the proposed method of medical watermarking attempts to provide guaranteed authenticity of transmitted medical information. The main advantages of the image watermarking for the medical applications are smaller storage space, reduced bandwidth requirement, confidentiality of the patient data and protection against tampering [1]. For tele-ophthalmology, tele-diagnosis and tele-consultancy services, medical images play a prominent role for instant diagnosis, understanding of crucial diseases as well as to avoid the misdiagnosis [2]. Currently, the combined methods of cryptography and watermarking have emerged to disseminate the security to the EPR medical data [3]. The main challenge for a good watermarking algorithm is robustness and security against the surviving attacks [4]. Any digital image consists of two important regions, region of interest (ROI) and non-region of interest (NROI). [5]. ROI is an area of image that has important data, so it cannot be allowed to be modified because most of the information is present in this area [6]. NROI is an area of image that does not have an important data i.e. background of image. The proper selection of an area of an image that does not have an important data for watermarking is crucial. It will give better protection if the data is embedded in NROI region of an image [7–9]. According to working domain method, the watermarking techniques can be classified as 'spatial domain' and 'transform domain' techniques [10]. To get robustness of watermarking technique transform domain watermarking is used. The reason of selecting transform domain is that it utilizes HVS features in a better way by spectral coefficients.

Various researchers have been proposed wavelet based watermarking to achieve higher robustness of hidden watermark [1, 11–17]. It includes space frequency localization, multi-resolution representation, multi-scale analysis, adaptability, linear complexity and support JPEG 2000. The overall performance of the wavelet based watermarking technique depends greatly on embedding and extraction process. The detail discussion of the DWT has been reported in Chap. 3.

The rest of the chapter is organized as follows. The related and recent state-of-the-art DWT based techniques are provided in Sect. 7.2. Section 7.3 provides the main contribution of the proposed work. The proposed technique is detailed in Sect. 7.4. The watermark embedding and extraction method is reported in Sects. 7.5 and 7.6, respectively. The experimental results and brief analysis of the work is reported in Sect. 7.7. Next, summary of the chapter is presented in Sect. 7.8.

7.2   Related Work

Various researchers have been proposed different watermarking techniques based on DWT and SVD [4, 18–20]. For a detailed description on these combined approaches, interested readers may directly refer to them. Kundu et al. [21] proposed a fragile watermarking technique with enhanced security and high payload embedding in spatial domain. A polygonal ROI is used to define diagnostic important part of image. EPR is encrypted by advanced encryption standard (AES) method by using secret key. After this the watermarked data is generated by compressing the payload data, which is defined by concatenating number of vertices in polygonal, vertex co-ordinates of ROI, hash of ROI generated by SHA-256, encrypted data and bits of ROI as binary string. Guo et al. [22] proposed a false positive free SVD based image watermarking scheme. It watermarked cover image by embedding the principal component of a watermark into the host image in block based manner using spread spectrum concept. Shuffled singular value decomposition (SSVD) is used in place of SVD to eliminate the false positive problem with wavelet transform domain to embed watermarks. Eswaraiah et al. [23] proposed a method of RONI watermarking with exact recovery of ROI using SHA-1. To authenticate ROI, Hash code of ROI is calculated using SHA-1 technique. After this it divided ROI and RONI in blocks considering that ROI has lesser number of pixels than RONI. The recovery data of each ROI block is embedded into LSBs of pixels inside the corresponding mapped RONI block.

Hajjaji et al. [24] proposed a medical image watermarking method based on DWT and K-L transform. The K-L transform applied only on details subbands of the second level DWT cover image. The visibility factor is determined by the fuzzy inference system. A binary signature owned by the hospital center is generated by SHA-1 hash function and the rest of patient record in a binary sequence concatenated with the binary signature. Before embedding the patient record into the cover image, it has been coded by the serial Turbo code. The method achieved high robustness and good imperceptibility against signal processing attacks.

Kannammal et al. [25] focused on the issue of the security for medical images and proposed an encryption based image watermarking method in frequency and spatial domain. The method using medical image as watermark and it is embedded in each block of cover image by altering the wavelet coefficients of chosen DWT subband. For the watermark embedding, least significant bit (LSB) method is used. After the embedding process, the watermarked image is encrypted by AES, RSA and RC4 algorithm and compared them. Based on the experimental results, RC4 encryption algorithm performs better than other two encryption algorithm. Also, the method achieved high robustness and security against signal processing attacks. Al-Haj et al. [26] presented a region based watermarking algorithm for medical images. The method used multiple watermarks in spatial (LSB) and frequency domain (DWT and SVD). With frequency domain techniques, robust watermarks embedded in region-of-non-interest (RONI) part of the cover image in order to avoid any compromise on its diagnostic value. However, fragile watermarks embed into region-of-interest (ROI) part of the image by using the spatial domain technique. The method achieved high robustness against JPEG and salt & pepper attacks. Badshah et al. [27] proposed a watermarking method based on Lempel-Ziv-Welch (LZW) compression technique using ultrasound medical images. In this method, the watermark is the combination of region of interest (ROI) and a secret key. The compression ratio has been compared with other compression techniques. Lu et al. [28] proposed a medical image watermarking algorithm using image and tag information as different watermarks. The image watermark is embedded in the ROI and the private tag information is embedded in the RONI part of the cover medical image. The watermark in the ROI is used to detect image tampering, and the watermark in the RONI is robust to different signal processing attacks.

7.3 Main Contribution of Work

The objective of this chapter is to develop a novel secure multiple text and image watermarking scheme on cover eye image using fusion of DWT and SVD for tele-ophthalmology application. Secure hash algorithm (SHA-512) is used for generating hash corresponding to iris part of the cover digital eye image and this unique hash parameter is used for enhancing the security feature of the proposed watermarking technique. Simultaneous embedding of four different watermarks (i.e. signature, index, caption and reference watermark) in form of image and text is embedding into the cover image. The suggested technique initially divides the digital eye image into ROI containing iris and NROI part where the text and image watermarks are embedded into the NROI part of the DWT cover image. The selection of DWT decomposition level for embedding the text and image watermarks depends on size, different characteristics and robustness requirements of medical watermark. The performance in terms of normalized correlation (NC) and bit error rate (BER) of the developed scheme is evaluated and analyzed against known signal processing attacks and 'Checkmark' attacks [29]. The proposed multilevel watermarking method correctly extracts the embedded watermarks without error and is robust against the all considered attacks without significant degradation of the medical image quality of the watermarked image. Therefore, the proposed method provides valuable solution for secure and compact medical data transmission for tele-ophthalmology applications. The following observations are apparent:

(i) *Fusion of DWT and SVD*: As discussed in chap. 3, the major advantages of DWT for watermarking applications are: space frequency localization, multi-resolution representation, multi-scale analysis, adaptability, linear complexity and compatible with JPEG 2000. Due to its excellent spatio-frequency localization properties, the DWT is also very suitable to determine the embedding areas in the cover image where a watermark can be imperceptibly embedded. One of attractive mathematical properties of SVD is that slight variations of singular values do not affect the visual perception of the cover image, which motivates the watermark embedding procedure to achieve better performance in terms of imperceptibility, robustness and capacity as compared to DWT and SVD applied individually. However, the main drawback of the SVD-based image watermarking is its false positive problem of which a specific watermark is detected in a watermarked image that actually was not embedded in it [22]. The false positive problem present in SVD can be removed by using shuffled SVD (SSVD) [22]. Shuffled SVD improves the reconstructed image quality by breaking an image into set of ensemble images. The Shuffled SVD can be viewed as a pre-processing from SVD by permuting the original image with the data-independent permutation. In the proposed method, shuffled SVD can be used in place of SVD to remove false positive problem.

(ii) *Improved performance*: The robustness of proposed method is compared with other reported techniques [30] and it is found that the proposed method offers superior performance. In addition, the method proposed by Singh et al. [30] has been embedded *812 bits* only. However, proposed method can embed *5145* bits with acceptable visual quality of the watermarked image (determined by PSNR values).

(iii) *Enhance security*: Security of the medical watermarks may be enhanced by using secure Hash Algorithm (SHA-512) [31, 32, 33]. MD5 (Message digest) and SHA-512 both are the hashing algorithm. In this research, the security of the watermark is the prime objective of the work. Table 7.1 [34] indicate the major differences between two hashing algorithms and show that SHA 512 is more secure than the MD5. However, the computational speed of the MD5 algorithm is faster than the SHA-512.

(iv) For identity authentication purposes, multiple watermarks are embedded instead of single watermark into the same medical image/multimedia objects simultaneously, which offer superior performance in tele-ophthalmology, tele-medicine and tele-diagnosis applications. In addition, simultaneous embed-ding of different watermarks on cover iris image while addressing the management of EPR data also.

(v) *Reduced storage and bandwidth requirements*: The medical image files/elec-tronic patient record (EPR) contain important patient data. Further, in order to conserve the transmission bandwidth or storage space the patient's details may be embedded inside the medical image.

Table 7.1 Comparison between two important hashing algorithms

Key points for comparison	MD5	SHA 512
Message-digest length in bits	128	512
Attack to try and find the original message given in message digest	Require 2^{128} operations to break in	require 2^{512} operations to break in, therefore more secure
Attack to try and find two message producing the same message digest	require 2^{64} operations to break in	require 2^{80} operations to break in
Speed	Faster (64 iterations, and 128-bit buffer)	Slower (80 iterations, and 512-bit buffer)
Software implementation	Simple	Simple

Table 7.2 Allocation of watermarks according to robustness and capacity criteria at different DWT sub-band

Sub-band used	Embedded watermark			Description of the considered watermarks
	Watermark types	Robustness requirements	Watermark size(bits)	
HL1	Reference	Low	512 × 512	Image watermark. To check the robustness against attacks
HL2	Caption	High	4480 bits	This watermark contains most of the part of patient information
HL3	Index	High	483 bits	It provides an index for each type of disease
LL4	Signature	Very high	182 bits	Smallest watermark. It contains physician's signature which is used for authentication purpose

7.4 Proposed Method

The proposed secure watermarking method provides a way of securing EPR data in cover eye image without affecting diagnostic important region (ROI). The selection of DWT decomposition level for embedding watermarks depends on size and desired robustness of watermark which is shown in Table 7.2.

The embedding of text and image watermarks is embedding in NROI part of the cover image. A medical image may contain several regions of interest but this proposed watermarking algorithm uses a single one. There are several ways of choosing ROI part of any medical image such as forming a square or polygonal [35, 36], defining a threshold [37], defining seeds [38, 39] etc. The proposed algorithm defines ROI part by forming a rectangular boundary. The wavelet domain ROI map is produced based on the spatial self similarity between sub-bands [40]. The ROI part of the cover Iris image is used for modifying text watermarks using SHA-512 which will enhance security feature of this medical image watermarking scheme [41].

The technique has four parts, the image watermark embedding and extraction processes, and the text watermark embedding and extraction processes. The details of the four algorithms are given in separate subsection:

7.5 Watermark Embedding Algorithms

The embedding of watermark can be divided in two parts: text watermark and image watermark. The cover image is first divided into two part ROI and NROI part. The DWT is applied on the NROI part of the cover image and now SVD is applied on the selected sub-band of the DWT cover. In addition, the hash value of the ROI part of the cover image is calculated by using the RSA hashing algorithm. The logical XOR operation has been applied on the ASCII value of the text watermark and the hash value of the ROI part of the cover which contain the encoded text watermark.

Finally, the image and encoded text watermark is embedded into the NROI part of the cover image. The detail description of the embedding algorithm for the text and image is given in Sects. 7.5.1 and 7.5.2 respectively. The extraction algorithm for the text and image is given in Sects. 7.6.1 and 7.6.2 respectively. The main steps of embedding these watermarks are given below:

1. Read the cover Iris image (*I*) of size (*M* × *N*).
2. Select iris by drawing a rectangular ROI for eye image and segment it,
3. Transform the image using "Haar" wavelet transform and get coefficients up to fourth level.
4. Apply SVD to selected sub-bands LL4, HL3, HL2 and HL1 which are used for embedding watermark.

7.5.1 Embedding Algorithm for Text Watermark

The embedding algorithm for text watermark is formulated as follows:

1. Read the message to be hidden and convert it into binary sequence.
2. Compute hash of ROI by using SHA-512 algorithm and convert it into binary sequence.
3. Perform a logical XOR operation between hash of ROI and binary sequence of watermark. This will give embedding watermark *w*.
4. Repeat above mentioned steps for generating encoded signature watermark w_s, index watermark w_i and caption watermark w_c.
5. Select singular values which belong to RONI randomly of subbands LL4, HL3 and HL2 according to the size of w_s, w_i and w_c respectively.
6. Replace these singular values by generated watermarks.
7. Generate respective subbands using these modified singular values and singular vectors of respective sub-bands.

7.5.2 Embedding Algorithm for Image Watermark

The embedding algorithm for image watermark is formulated as follows:

1. Read the image watermark 'w_{im}' size equal to size of sub band HL1.
2. Apply SVD to HL1 and 'w_{im}' to compute singular values of them. Let singular values for HL1 and 'w_{im}' are λ_c and λ_w respectively.
3. Modify singular value in HL1 subband by the equation (7.1):

$$\lambda_{cw} = \lambda_c + (\alpha \times \lambda_w) \tag{7.1}$$

Where α is a scale factor.

4. Generate HL1 with this modified singular value.

5. Take inverse DWT to generate watermarked image.
6. Add ROI part to the watermarked image.

7.6 Watermark Extraction Algorithm

For extracting watermarks, we used the same hash of ROI and embedding key to extract watermark. To generate original watermarks cover image and original reference image is also required to get singular value. Following steps are applied to extract the watermark:

7.6.1 Extraction Algorithm for Text Watermark

The extraction algorithm for text watermark is formulated as follows:

1. Transform watermarked image using "Haar" wavelet transform and get coefficients up to fourth level.
2. Apply SVD to 4th level approximation coefficients a_4, 3rd level horizontal coefficients b_3 and 2nd level horizontal coefficients b_2.
3. Using same random pattern of selection of singular value generate the embedded watermarks bit by following equation for each above mentioned levels:

$$t_{ext} = \lambda_{wm} - \lambda_o \tag{7.2}$$

4. Here λ_{wm} and λ_o are singular values of watermarked subbands and cover image subbands respectively.
5. Perform logical XOR operation between t_{ext} and hash of ROI which gives binary sequence of extracted watermark.
6. Convert these extracted binary sequences to character to generate original text watermark.

7.6.2 Extraction Algorithm for Image Watermark

The extraction algorithm for image watermark is formulated as follows:

1. Apply SVD to 1st level horizontal coefficients b_1.
2. Compute singular value for extracted image watermark by following equation:

$$\lambda_{ext} = (\lambda_{cw} - \lambda_c) / \alpha \tag{7.3}$$

3. Generate extracted image watermark using this singular value λ_{ext} and singular vectors of original reference image watermark which will give extracted reference watermark.

7.7   Experimental Results and Performance Analysis

The performance of the proposed multiple watermarking technique is based on DWT, SVD and secure Hash Algorithm (SHA-512) is investigated. The text watermarks are extracted successfully from watermarked image using embedding key and hash of ROI of eye image. In the proposed method cover image of size 1024 × 1024, the image watermark of size 512 × 512 considered as a reference watermark and the text watermark of varying size are used for testing. The robustness of the image and text watermarks is evaluated by determining NC and BER respectively. The quality of the watermarked image is evaluated by PSNR. It is quite apparent that size of the watermark affects quality of the watermarked image. The size of the watermark is sum total of bits occupied by all watermarks in the case of multiple watermarking. However, degradation in quality of the watermarked image will not be observable if the size of watermark (total size in case of multiple watermarking) is small. Figure 7.1a, b shows the cover and watermarked image respectively. Figure 7.2 show the extracted signature, index and caption watermarks. Figure 7.3a, b shows original and extracted reference watermarks respectively.

Table 7.3 shows the PSNR, BER and NC performance of the proposed method at different scale factor. It is found that larger gain factor results in stronger robustness of the extracted watermark whereas smaller gain factor provides better PSNR values between original and watermarked medical images. The maximum PSNR value is 35.84 dB and BER = 0 against at gain factor = 0.01. Here, the NC value is 0.8 However, the maximum NC value is 0.99 at gain factor = 0.2. Here, the PSNR value is 39.97 dB. For all the considered text watermark BER value is Zero. It is found that larger the gain factor results stronger robustness of extracting watermark whereas smaller the gain factor provides better visual quality of the watermarked image.

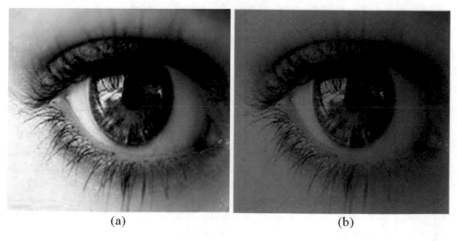

(a)   (b)

Fig. 7.1 Image (**a**) cover eye and (**b**) watermarked

Doctor Signature: Dr. Anoop Chauhan (MBBS, MD)
Disease Type: C71.7 Brain Stem: Fourth ventricle, Infratentorial NOS ICD-10
STANDARDS
Patient Information:
Patient Name: Ravindra Srivastava
Patient Age: 50 Years
Patient Address: 213/54 HIG Colony Block B, Krishnapuram Kanpur
Doctor Name: Dr. Anoop Chauhan (MBBS, MD)
Medical Centre: Doctor Chauhan eye centre, ISO Certified eye hospital
Affiliation: BBS Memorial Charitable Hospital Society
CMO Registration Number: 1234/2345
First Visit Date: 3/12/15
Problem Diagnosed: Improper Vision, Clotting of Blood
Second Visit Date: 5/12/15
Right eye axis: 20' Left eye axis: 70'
Right eye vision: 6/6 Left eye vision: 7/7
Testing: Vision Test, Corneal and Retinal Topography
Suggestion by Doctor: Refractive Surgery

Fig. 7.2 Extracted Signature, Index and Caption watermark

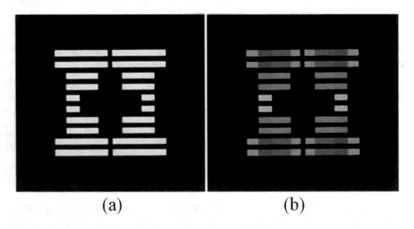

(a)   (b)

Fig. 7.3 Reference (**a**) original and (**b**) extracted watermark

Table 7.3 PSNR, BER and NC performance at different factor

Scale factor (α)	PSNR (dB)	BER values for text watermark			NC values for image watermark
		Signature watermark	Index watermark	Caption watermark	
0.01	54.26	0	0	0	0.87
0.03	51.79	0	0	0	0.91
0.05	48.42	0	0	0	0.93
0.07	45.82	0	0	0	0.96
0.09	42.68	0	0	0	0.98
0.2	39.97	0	0	0	0.99

In this study, JPEG attacks with different quality factors are considered as signal a processing attack which is shown in Table 7.4. However, the other attacks are considered as Checkmark attacks which is shown in Table 7.5. Table 7.4 shows BER and NC performance of the proposed method for JPEG attacks at different quality factors (QF) at gain = 0.09. The highest NC value of 0.98 has been obtained against JPEG Compression with quality factor = 95. However, the minimum NC value of 0.957 has been obtained against JPEG Compression with quality factor = 55. For the entire considered text watermark BER value is Zero. Table 7.5 shows the BER and NC performance of the proposed method for 'Checkmark' attacks. The maximum BER value of 8.514 has been obtained against Gaussian Noise (Mean = 0, Variance = 0.05) for the caption watermark, where the NC value is 0.792. However, the maximum NC value of 0.99 has been obtained against Flip, where the BER value is '0' for the entire chosen text watermark.

In Table 7.6, the visual quality (determined by PSNR values) of the watermarked image robustness performance (determined NC values) of the proposed method is compared with other methods [30] at different gain factors. It is observed that the

Table 7.4 BER and NC performance for JPEG attacks at different quality factors (QF)

| JPEG attacks | BER values for text watermark | | | NC values for image watermark |
	Signature watermark	Index watermark	Caption watermark	
QF = 95	0	0	0	0.98
QF = 85	0	0	0	0.975
QF = 75	0	0	0	0.964
QF = 65	0	0	0	0.96
QF = 55	0	0	0	0.957

Table 7.5 BER and NC performance for 'Checkmark' attacks

| Checkmark attacks | BER values for text watermark | | | NC values for image watermark |
	Signature watermark	Index watermark	Caption watermark	
Sharpening	0	0	0	0.918
Gaussian Noise (Mean = 0, Variance = 0.01)	0	0	0	0.8325
Gaussian Noise (Mean = 0, Variance = 0.05)	0	1.62	8.514	0.792
Frequency mode LR Attack	0	0	0	0.6628
Flip	0	0	0	0.99
Median Filtering [2 2] and [3 3]	0	0	0	0.9077 and 0.8560
Hard threshold	0	0	0	0.9834
Rotation(20°)	0	0	0	0.9255
Dither	0	0	0	0.7058
Scaling by 2.5	0	1.01	6.45	0.695
Warping (wf = 5)	0	0	0	0.624
Wiener Filtering [2 2] and [3 3]	0	0	0	0.9125 and 0.862

Table 7.6 Comparison of PSNR and NC values with other reported method

Gain factor	Singh et al. [30]		Proposed method	
	PSNR (dB)	NC	PSNR (dB)	NC
0.01	28.17	0.5247	54.26	0.87
0.05	28.02	0.9288	48.42	0.93
0.09	217	0.9668	42.68	0.98
0.1	26.85	0.9697	39.58	0.984

proposed method offers higher visual quality and robustness at all considered gain as compared to the other reported method. Referring this table, the maximum NC value with proposed method has been obtained as 0.984 against 0.9697 obtained by Singh et al. in [30] method at gain factor = 0.1. However, the minimum NC value with proposed method has been obtained as 0.87 against 0.5247 obtained by Singh et al. in [30] method at gain factor = 0.01. The maximum PSNR value has been obtained with Singh et al. in [30] is 28.17 dB. However, the maximum PSNR value has been obtained by the proposed method is 54.26 dB at gain factor = 0.01. However, the minimum PSNR value has been obtained with Singh et al. in [30] is 26.85 dB. However, the minimum PSNR value has been obtained by the proposed method is 39.58 dB at gain factor = 0.1. In addition, the method proposed by Singh et al. [30] has been embedded 812 bits only. However, in our proposed method, we can embed 5145 bits with the acceptable PSNR performance. Overall, the performance of the proposed method is better than the other reported technique [30] in terms of robustness, capacity and security. Finally, the overall PSNR, NC and BER performance of the proposed method highly depends on the size of the watermarks (image and text), gain factor and the noise variation.

7.8 Summary

The proposed algorithm provided a new watermarking technique for eye care centers dealing with eye image transmission by hiding information about patient and doctor in a secure way using cryptographic hash function of the iris pattern. Each embedded watermarks has different characteristics in terms of capacity, type and size of information, robustness and application. The described watermarking technique is robust to compression and 'Checkmark' attacks. Use of SVD along with DWT increased the robustness of algorithm. As the hash encoded watermarks were embedded randomly in singular values hence without knowledge of embedding key, data could not be extracted which enhanced the security of watermarking system. In this research, the gray scale images have been considered. However, the watermark embedding into colour image provides greater space against the watermark embedding into gray scale image. This space will hide more watermark information (capacity will improve). The choice of colour space and selection of embedding color channel is important 'RGB' model and watermarking in blue plane is not suitable due to poor robustness against compression attacks. This is because the blue channel is heavily quantized during JPEG compression. However, blue channel is able to give better imperceptibility. The 'YCbCr' model gives advantage of robustness against compression attacks if watermark is embedded in 'Y' channel because 'Y' channel is less quantized as compared to chrominance channels ('Cb' and 'Cr') in JPEG compression process. However, 'Y' channel (Luminance) is more sensitive to human eyes. Therefore, even small modifications in the wavelet coefficients of this channel may lead to poor imperceptibility which limits the embedding capacity of 'Y' channel. The major findings of this work is identified as follows:

(i) With excellent spatio-frequency localization properties, the DWT is also very suitable to determine the embedding areas in the cover image where a watermark can be imperceptibly embedded. One of attractive mathematical properties of SVD is that slight variations of singular values do not affect the visual perception of the cover image, which motivates the watermark embedding procedure to achieve better performance in terms of imperceptibility, robustness and capacity as compared to DWT and SVD applied individually.

(ii) For identity authentication purposes, multiple watermarks are embedded instead of single watermark into the same medical image/multimedia objects simultaneously, which offer superior performance in medical applications.

(iii) The PSNR and NC performance of the proposed method is compared with other reported techniques and it is found that the proposed method offers superior performance. In addition, the capacity of embedding text watermarks is better than the other reported technique.

(iv) Security of the medical watermarks is enhanced by using secure Hash Algorithm (SHA-512) for generating hash of ROI part (iris) of the cover eye image, which provides 256 bits of hash.

(v) The medical image files/electronic patient record (EPR) contain important patient data. Further, in order to conserve the transmission bandwidth or storage space the patient's details may be embedded inside the medical image.

(vi) The proposed multilevel watermarking approach aims to simultaneously embed different types of watermarks on cover eye image while addressing the management of EPR data also.

This method may provide a potential solution to existing tele-ophthalmology security problem of patient identity theft. The inclusions of many techniques were combined to improve the robustness, high capacity (in form of multiple watermarks) and include the security of the watermarks with the acceptable quality of the watermarked image for the tele-ophthalmology application which is the prime objective of the research. However, it may have increased the computational complexity to some extent which needs to be investigated separately.

We would like to further improve the performance in terms of robustness, visual quality of the watermarked image, additional security of watermark, capacity of the cover multimedia object, false positive problem of the SVD and poor directionality information of DWT, which will be reported in future communication.

References

1. A.K. Singh, M. Dave, A. Mohan, Hybrid technique for robust and imperceptible multiple watermarking using medical images. J. Multimedia Tools Appl. **75**(14), 8381–8401 (2016)
2. C. Rey, J.L. Dugelay, A survey of watermarking algorithm for image authentication. EURASIP J. Appl. Signal Process. **2002**(1), 613–621 (2002)
3. S.M. Mousavi, A. Naghsh, S.A.R. Abu-Bakar, Watermarking techniques used in medical images: a survey. J. Digit. Imaging **27**(6), 714–729 (2014)
4. A.K. Singh, B. Kumar, M. Dave, A. Mohan, Robust and imperceptible dual watermarking for telemedicine applications. Wirel. Pers. Commun. **80**(4), 1415–1433 (2015)
5. A.K. Singh, M. Dave, A. Mohan, Wavelet based image watermarking: futuristic concepts in information security. Proc. Natl. Acad. Sci., India Sect. A: Phys. Sci. **84**(3), 345–359 (2014)
6. L. Zhang, P.-P. Zhou, Localized affine transform resistant watermarking in region-of-interest. Telecommun. Syst. **44**(3), 205–220 (2010)
7. C.-Y. Yang, W.-C. Hu, Reversible data hiding in the spatial and frequency domains. Int. J. Image Process. **3**(6), 373–384 (2010)
8. J. Zain, M. Clarke, Security in telemedicine: issue in watermarking medical images, in Proceedings of 3rd International Conference on Science of Electronic, Technologies of Information and Telecommunications, TUNISIA, 27–31 Mar 2005
9. N.A. Memon, S.A.M. Gilani, NROI watermarking of medical images for content authentication, in Proceedings of 12th IEEE International Multi Topic Conference, Karachi, Pakistan, pp. 106–110, 2008
10. A.K. Singh, Some new techniques of improved wavelet domain watermarking for medical images, Ph.D. Thesis, National Institute of Technology Kurukshetra, Haryana, India, 2015
11. C.-C. Lai, C.-C. Tsai, Digital image watermarking using discrete wavelet transform and singular value decomposition. IEEE Trans. Instrum. Meas. **59**(11), 3060–3063 (2010)
12. K. Pal, G. Ghosh, M. Bhattacharya, Biomedical image watermarking in wavelet domain for data integrity using bit majority algorithm and multiple copies of hidden information. Am. J. Biomed. Eng. **2**(2), 29–37 (2012)
13. A.K. Singh, M. Dave, A. Mohan, Multilevel encrypted text watermarking on medical images using spread-spectrum in DWT domain. Wirel. Pers. Commun. **83**(3), 2133–2150 (2015)
14. W.-H. Lin, Y.-R. Wang, S.-J. Horng, T.-W. Kao, P. Yi, A blind watermarking method using maximum wavelet coefficient quantization. Expert Syst. Appl. **36**(9), 11509–11516 (2009)
15. W.-H. Lin, Y.-R. Wang, S.-J. Horng, A wavelet-tree-based watermarking method using distance vector of binary cluster. Expert Syst. Appl. **36**(6), 9869–9878 (2009)
16. W.-H. Lin, S.-J. Horng, T.-W. Kao, P. Fan, C.-L. Lee, P. Yi, An efficient watermarking method based on significant difference of wavelet coefficient quantization. IEEE Trans. Multimedia **10**(5), 746–757 (2008)
17. A.K. Singh, B. Kumar, M. Dave, A. Mohan, Multiple watermarking on medical images using selective DWT coefficients. J. Med. Imaging Health Inf. **5**(3), 607–614 (2015)
18. R. Dhanalakshmi, K. Thaiyalnayaki, Dual watermarking scheme with encryption. Int. J. Computer Sci. Inf. Security **7**(1), 248–253 (2010)
19. L.H. Mahajan, S.A. Patil, Image watermarking scheme using SVD. Int. J. Adv. Res. Sci. Eng. **2**(6), 69–77 (2013)
20. C.-C. Lai, C.-C. Tsai, Digital image watermarking using discrete wavelet transform and singular value decomposition. IEEE Trans. Instrum. Meas. **59**(11), 3060–3063 (2010)
21. Kundu, M. Kumar, S. Das, Lossless ROI medical image watermarking technique with enhanced security and high payload embedding, 20th International Conference on Pattern Recognition (ICPR), Istanbul, Turkey, pp. 1457–1460, August 2010
22. J.-M. Guo, H. Prasetyo, False-positive-free SVD-based image watermarking. J. Vis. Commun. Image Represent. **25**(5), 1149–1163 (2014)
23. R. Eswaraiah, E. Sreenivasa Reddy, Medical image watermarking technique for accurate tamper detection in ROI and exact recovery of ROI. Int. J. Telemed. Appl. **2014**, 1–10 (2014)

24. M.A. Hajjaji, E.-B. Bourennane, A.B. Abdelali, A. Mtibaa, Combining Haar Wavelet and Karhunen Loeve transforms for medical images watermarking. Biomed. Res. Int. **2014**, 1–15 (2014)
25. A. Kannammal, S. Subha Rani, Two level security for medical images using watermarking/encryption algorithms. Int. J. Imaging Syst. Technol. **24**, 111–120 (2014)
26. A. Al-Haj, A. Amer, Secured telemedicine using region-based watermarking with tamper localization. J. Digit. Imaging **27**(6), 737–750 (2014)
27. G. Badshah, S.-C. Liew, J.M. Zain, M. Ali, Watermark compression in medical image watermarking using lempel-ziv-welch (LZW) lossless compression technique. J. Digit. Imaging **29**, 216–225 (2015)
28. J. Lu, M. Wang, J. Dai, Q. Huang, L. Li, C.-C. Chang, Multiple watermark scheme based on DWT-DCT quantization for medical images. J. Inf. Hiding Multimedia Signal Process. Ubiquitous Int. **6**(3), 458–472 (2015)
29. S. Pereira, S. Voloshynovskiy, M. Madueño, S. Marchand-Maillet, T. Pun, Second generation benchmarking and application oriented evaluation, in Information Hiding Workshop III, Pittsburgh, PA, USA, pp. 340–353, 2001
30. A.K. Singh, M. Dave, A. Mohan, Robust and secure multiple watermarking in wavelet domain. A special issue on advanced signal processing technologies and systems for healthcare applications (ASPTSHA). J. Med. Imaging Health Inf. **5**(2), 606–614 (2015)
31. C. Paar, J. Pelzl, *Understanding Cryptography: A Textbook for Students and Practitioners*, 3rd edn. (Springer, New York, 2009), pp. 29–53
32. D. Bouslimi, G. Coatrieux, M. Cozic, C. Roux, A joint encryption/watermarking system for verifying the reliability of medical images. IEEE Trans. Inf. Technol. Biomed. **16**, 891–899 (2012)
33. P.W. Wong, N. Memon, Secret and public key image watermarking scheme for image authentication and ownership verification. IEEE Trans. Image Process. **10**(10), 1593–1601 (2001)
34. A. Kahate, *Cryptography and Network Security*, 3rd edn. (TMH, New York, 2013)
35. G. Aggeliki, S. Pavlopoulos, D. Koutsouris, Secure and efficient health data management through multiple watermarking on medical images. Med. Biol. Eng. Comput. **44**(8), 619–631 (2006)
36. J.M. Zain, M. Clarke, Reversible region of non-interest (RONI) watermarking for authentication of DICOM images. Int. J. Computer Sci. Network Security **7**(9), 19–28 (2007)
37. S. Das, M.K. Kundu, Effective management of medical information through ROI-lossless fragile image watermarking technique. Comput. Methods Prog. Biomed. **111**(3), 662–675 (2013)
38. B.L. Gunjal, S.N. Mali, ROI based embedded watermarking of medical images for secured communication in telemedicine. Int. J. Computer Commun. Eng. **6**(48), 293–298 (2012)
39. K. Pal, V.H. Mankar, T.S. Das, S.K. Sarkar, Contour detection and recovery through bio-medical watermarking for telediagnosis. Int. J. Tomograph. Simul. **14**(S10), 109–119 (2010)
40. P.C. Su, H.J. Wang, C.C.J. Kuo, Digital image watermarking in regions of interest, in Proceedings of 1999 PICS 52nd Annual Conference Savannah, Georgia, pp. 295–300, 1999
41. F. Ahmed, M.Y. Siyal, V.U. Abbas, A secure and robust hash-based scheme for image authentication. Signal Process. **90**(5), 1456–1470 (2010)

Chapter 8
Secure Multiple Watermarking Technique Using Neural Networks

Amit Kumar Singh, Basant Kumar, Ghanshyam Singh, and Anand Mohan

8.1 Introduction

The continuous developments in information and communication technologies (ICTs) and multimedia technology offers widespread use of multimedia contents such as images, audio and video [1]. All these technological advancements introduced a progressive change in various health care facilities such as information management, Hospital Information System (HIS), medical imaging and health social networks [1, 2]. Telemedicine is defined as use of ICTs in order to provide healthcare services when practicing doctors, patients and researchers are present in different geographical locations [3]. Although such transmission and distribution of electronic patient record (EPR) raises security related issues such as reliability, integrity, security, authenticity and confidentiality [4–7]. In recent years, the watermarking technology is a value added tools for different health data management

A.K. Singh (✉)
Department of Computer Science & Engineering, Jaypee University of Information
Technology, Waknaghat, Solan, India
e-mail: amit_245singh@yahoo.com

B. Kumar
Department of Electronics and Communication Engineering, Motilal Nehru National
Institute of Technology, Allahabad, India
e-mail: singhbasant@yahoo.com

G. Singh
Department of Electronics and Communication Engineering, Jaypee University
of Information Technology, Waknaghat, Solan, India
e-mail: drghanshyam.singh@yahoo.com

A. Mohan
Department of Electronics Engineering,
Indian Institute of Technology (BHU), Varanasi, India
e-mail: profanandmohan@gmail.com

© Springer International Publishing AG 2017
A.K. Singh et al. (eds.), *Medical Image Watermarking*, Multimedia Systems
and Applications, DOI 10.1007/978-3-319-57699-2_8

issues [5, 6] and medical identity theft in healthcare applications [8–11] to involve hiding information within the cover data and the hidden information can be later recovered at the receiver side for purposes of ownership verification, unique authentication. Despite the extensive literature on wide range of applications, some researcher/scientist has been reported little work toward the development of health-oriented perspectives of watermarking [5, 6, 12–21]. Robustness, imperceptibility, capacity, computational cost and security are important benchmark parameters for general watermarking system [11]. Various noted researcher/scientist strive to developed different watermarking techniques for improving one or a subset of these parameters [12–15, 20, 21]. However, it is noticed that they compromise with other remaining parameters. Thus, there is need to develop effective watermarking methods that can offer good trade-off between these benchmark parameters. The proposed research/work presented in the chapter is focuses on to optimize trade-off between these benchmark parameters. Therefore, some optimization techniques are required to balance these benchmark parameters. Recently, Artificial Intelligence (AI) techniques such as genetic algorithm (GA), differential evolution (DE), neural networks (NN), Clonal selection algorithm (CSA) and particle swarm optimizer (PSO) [22–27] are used as an optimization technique to search optimal sub-bands and coefficients in transform domain to embed watermark with different scaling factors. In addition, these techniques can be used as optimization techniques to remove some round off errors when coefficients in transform domain are transformed to spatial domain.

The rest of the chapter is organized as follows. The related and recent state-of-the-art DWT based techniques are provided in Sect. 8.2. Section 8.3 provides the main contribution of the proposed work. The proposed technique is detailed in Sect. 8.4. The experimental results and brief analysis of the work is reported in Sect. 8.5. Next, our summary of the chapter is presented in Sect. 8.6

8.2 Related Work

A brief review of recent and related watermarking methods using DWT is presented below:

In [4], the authors present a multiple watermarking method using combination of DWT and SVD. Further, the method enhanced the security and robustness of the watermark information, encryption and Reed-Solomon ECC is applied to the watermark before embedding into the cover medical image. The method is robust for different attacks including the Checkmark attacks. Yen et al. [27] presents a digital watermarking using DCT and BPNN. In the embedding process, DCT has been applied on the cover image of size 256×256 and the watermark of size 32×32 is embedded into the mid frequency region of the cover. The simulation results indicated that the method is found to be robust for different attacks. Ganic and Eskicioglu [28] presents a hybrid method based on DWT and Singular Value Decomposition (SVD). In the embedding process, the singular values of all DWT cover sub-band information are modified with singular values of watermark information. The method is robust for different known attacks. Terzija et al. [29] proposed a method for improving the efficiency and robustness of the image watermarks using three different error correction codes (ECCs). Out of the three ECCs, Reed-Solomon code performs better than the BCH and Hamming code. The experimental results show that the method is robust for different attacks. However, the method unable to correct the error rates greater than 20%. A DWT-SVD based image watermarking method is presented by Lai et al. [30], where the watermark information is directly embedded into the singular vector of the cover image's DWT sub-bands. The experimental results show that the method is robust for different known attacks at acceptable visual quality of the watermarked image.

Vafaei et al. [31] proposed a blind watermarking method using DWT and Feed forward Neural Networks (FNN). In the embedding process, third level DWT applied on cover image and divides the selected sub-bands into different blocks. To enhance the robustness of the proposed method, the binary watermark information is embedded repetitively into the selected DWT coefficients. Experimental results demonstrate that the proposed method offer good visual quality of the watermarked image and robust against different kinds of signal processing attacks. Ali et al. [32] proposed a watermarking scheme based on Differential Evolution using DWT and SVD. In the embedding process, the singular vector of selected DWT sub-band of the cover is modified with binary watermark image. The proposed method claimed that it offer the solution for false positive problem as suffer by SVD. Mehto et al. [33] proposed a medical image watermarking using DWT and DCT. The watermark image contains patient information is embedded in to the medical cover image. The performance of the method is evaluated for different gain without using any attacks. Nguyen et al. [34] proposed reversible watermarking method using DWT. In this method, an authentication code is randomly generated and embedded into DWT sub-bands of each image block. The method is extensively evaluated for different kinds of attacks including tampered regions of different sizes, content tampered attack and collage attack. In addition, some important image watermarking techniques using neural networks have been proposed [35–37]. For a detailed description on these approaches, interested readers may directly refer to them.

8.3 Important Contribution of the Work

This chapter presents a hybrid approach (DWT, DCT and SVD) for multilevel watermarking of medical images using BPNN. The proposed method is based on popular transform domain techniques so their fusion makes a very attractive watermarking technique. Due to its excellent spatio-frequency localization properties, the DWT is very suitable to identify areas in the cover image where a watermark can be imperceptibly embedded [21, 38, 39]. However, DWT is shift sensitive, poor directionality information and lacks the phase information [39]. DCT has good energy compaction property. However, one of the main problems and the criticism of the

DCT is the blocking effect [39, 40]. An attractive mathematical property of SVD is that slight variations of singular values do not affect the visual quality of the cover medical image, which motivates the watermark embedding procedure to achieve better performance in terms of imperceptibility, robustness and capacity as compared to DWT, DCT and SVD applied individually. However, one of the main drawbacks of the SVD-based image watermarking is its false positive problem [39]. The false positive problem present in SVD is addressing in some reported techniques [41, 42]. The important contribution of the work is summarized below:

1. *Enhanced the capacity and security of watermarks*: In this method, multiple watermarks (text and image) are embedded simultaneously, which provides extra level of security with acceptable PSNR, BER and NC performance. For identity authentication purposes, multiple watermarks have been embedded instead of single watermark into the same cover medical image/multimedia objects simultaneously, which offer superior performance (extra level of security) in healthcare applications. However, the embedding of multiple watermarks in the same multimedia object decreases the PSNR performance and increase the computational time. Security of the Lump image watermark is enhanced by using Arnold transform before embedding into the cover. In addition, a popular lossless compression technique (arithmetic coding) is applied to symptoms watermark to compress the size of the watermark. This compression techniques can correctly recovered all bits of the symptom watermark in lossless manner. The signature watermark containing doctor's identification code for the purpose of origin authentication is embedding into the higher level DWT sub-band. In order to increase the robustness of the signature watermark and reduce the channel distortion, Hamming error correcting code is applied to the watermark before embedding into the cover.

2. *Improved the robustness of image and text watermark*: Tables 8.2, 8.3, 8.4, 8.5, 8.6 shows the effect of Back Propagation Neural Network (BPNN) [43] which offers higher robustness compared to without using the BPNN. In this neural network process, each input layer node is connected to a node from hidden layer and the hidden layer node is connected to a node in output layer. Further, the input layer is duplicated every single input and sends down to the hidden layer nodes. The hidden layer uses input values and modifies them using some weight value, this modified value is than send to the next layer (output) but it will also be modified by some weight from connection between hidden and output layer. Finally, the output layer process information received from its previous layer and produces output, which is processed by activation function. In addition, the robustness (reduce BER values) of the text watermark is also enhanced by using the Hamming ECC.

3. *Save the storage and bandwidth requirements*: Embedding patient's information in form of the multiple watermarks (image and text both) in cover images conserves transmission bandwidth and storage space requirements, and

4. The proposed method addressing the health data management issues also [6].

8.4   Proposed Algorithm

The proposed multilevel watermarking of medical images embeds multiple water-marks in the form of text and image into medical cover image. Table 8.1 shows the allocation of image and text watermarks according to robustness and capacity retire-ments at different DWT sub-bands. It is evident that watermarks containing impor-tant information and requiring more robustness are embedded in higher level DWT sub-bands [3, 4, 7].

In this method, multiple image and text watermarks are embedded in the medical cover image. In the embedding process, the cover medical image is decomposed into third-level DWT. Low-high frequency band (LH1) of the first level DWT is transformed by DCT and then SVD is applied to DCT coefficients. The image watermark is also transformed by DCT and SVD. The singular values of the water-mark image information are embedded in the singular value of the cover medical image. The image, symptom and signature watermark is embedded in to the first (LH1), second (LH2) and third level (LL3) DWT sub-band of the cover image respectively. Further, Lump watermark is scrambled by using Arnold transform before embedding into the cover which provides the extra level of security. Moreover, the symptom and signature text watermarks are also compressed/encoded by lossless arithmetic compression technique (for embedding more information and can recovered all watermark bits in lossless manner) and Hamming error correction code (for improving the robustness and reducing the channel distortion) respec-tively. The compressed and encoded text watermarks are then embedded into the cover image. Results are obtained by varying the gain factor, text watermark size and the different cover image modalities. Experimental results are provided to illus-trate that the proposed method is able to withstand a known attacks. The proposed algorithm has two different parts, the embedding and extraction process. Figure 8.1a, b shows the proposed method for embedding and extraction process respectively. The image watermark embedding and extraction process are given in sections 8.4.1 and 8.4.2 respectively. However, the text watermarks embedding and extraction pro-cess [29] are given in sections 8.4.3 and 8.4.4 respectively.

Table 8.1 Allocation of different watermarks according to robustness and capacity criteria at different sub-band

SN	Medical watermark	DWT sub band	Purpose of embedding
1	Signature	LL3	Contains Doctor's Identification code for the purpose of Authentication
2	Symptoms	LH2	Contains Patient's history and diagnostic reports related information for the purpose of preventing addition storage, transmission requirements and in order to increase capacity
3	Lump	LH1	Contains reference image watermark for the purpose of data integrity control

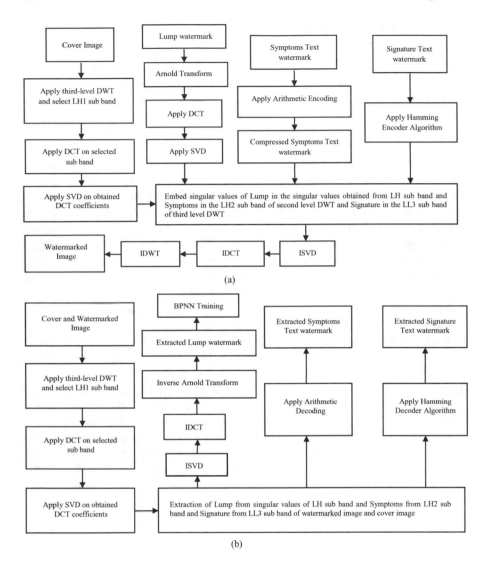

Fig. 8.1 Watermark (**a**) embedding and (**b**) extraction process

8.4.1 Embedding Algorithm for Image Watermark

1. Apply third-level DWT transform on cover image to decompose it into corresponding sub bands and select LH1 sub-band.
2. Apply DCT to the selected sub-band and then apply SVD to transformed DCT coefficients to obtain corresponding three matrices U, S and V.

$$A_c = U_c S_c V_c^T \tag{8.1}$$

3. Encrypt the Lump watermark image using Arnold Transform
4. Apply DCT on encrypted Lump watermark image and then apply SVD to DCT coefficients to obtain corresponding matrices similar to step 2.

$$A_w = U_w S_w V_w^T \qquad (8.2)$$

5. Modify the singular values of LH1 sub band of cover image with the singular values of Lump.

$$S_{wat} = S_c + k \times S_w \qquad (8.3)$$

Here 'k' is defined as the scaling/gain factor with which watermark images are embedded into host image.

6. Obtain modified DCT coefficients by applying Inverse Singular Value Decomposition (ISVD) using following equations.

$$A_{wat} = U_c \times S_{wat} \times V_c^T \qquad (8.4)$$

7. Obtain modified LH1* sub band by applying Inverse Discrete Cosine Transform (IDCT) to modified DCT coefficients.
8. Change LH1 sub band of cover image with the modified LH1* sub band and apply Inverse Discrete Wavelet Transform (IDWT) to get watermarked image.
9. Apply attacks and noise to the watermarked image to check the robustness of the proposed algorithm.

8.4.2 Extraction Algorithm for Image Watermark

1. Apply third-level DWT transform on cover image to decompose it into corresponding sub bands and select LH1 sub band.
2. Apply DCT to the selected sub-band and then apply SVD to transformed DCT coefficients to obtain their corresponding three matrices U, S and V.

$$A_c = U_c S_c V_c^T \qquad (8.5)$$

3. Apply DCT on watermark image (Lump) and then apply SVD to DCT coefficients to obtain their corresponding matrices similar to step 2.

$$A_w = U_w S_w V_w^T \qquad (8.6)$$

4. Apply step 1, step 2 to watermarked image to obtain its corresponding SVD Matrices for LH1 sub band.

$$A_{wat} = U_{wat}S_{wat}V_{wat}{}^{T}$$ (8.7)

5. Obtain singular values of Lump from the singular values of LH1 sub band of watermarked image and cover image respectively by using following equation:

$$S_w{}^* = (S_{wat} - S_c)/\text{gain}(k)$$ (8.8)

6. Obtain extracted watermark by applying inverse singular value decomposition (ISVD) using equation (9) and then inverse discrete Cosine transform (IDCT).

$$A_{ew} = U_w \times S_w{}^* \times V_w{}^{T}$$ (8.9)

7. Decrypt the extracted watermark by applying inverse Arnold Transform to obtain final extracted Lump image watermark
8. BPNN is then applied to extracted watermarks to remove noise and interferences in order to improve their robustness. Figure 8.2 shows the BPNN training process.

8.4.3 Embedding Algorithm for Text Watermark

Text watermarks (Signature and Symptoms) are embedded into cover image [29] using following steps:

1. Apply third-level DWT transform on cover image to decompose it into corresponding sub bands and select LH2 and LL3 sub bands.
2. Convert the Signature text watermark into binary bits.
3. Apply Hamming encoder algorithm to binary bits of Signature text watermark and replace (0, 1) by (−1, 1) in the watermarking bits.
4. Apply Arithmetic Encoding to Symptoms text watermark and replace (0, 1) by (−1, 1) in the watermarking bits similar to step3.
5. Embed the text watermarking bits obtained from Symptoms watermark to LH2 sub band of cover image and watermarking bits obtained from Signature watermark to LL3 sub band of cover image using equation.

$$A_i'(x,y) = A_i(x,y)(1 + k \times Wbt_i);$$ (8.10)

Where, i = Signature and Symptoms text watermarks.
$A_i'(x,y)$ and $A(x,y)$ are DWT coefficients before and after embedding process, Wbt_i is text watermarking bits and 'k' is the gain factor.

6. Change LH2 and LL3 sub bands of cover image with the modified LH2* and LL3*sub band and apply IDWT to get watermarked image.

Fig. 8.2 BPNN training process [39]

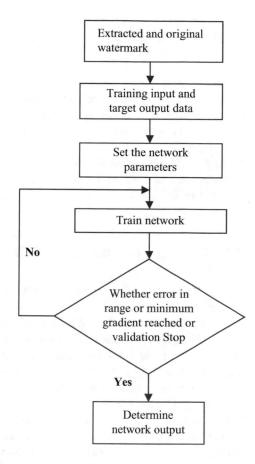

8.4.4 Extraction Algorithm for Text Watermark

Text watermarks (Signature and Symptoms) are extracted [29] from watermarked image using following steps: -

1. Apply third-level DWT transform on cover image to decompose it into corresponding sub bands and select LH2 and LL3 sub bands.
2. Apply third-level DWT transform on watermarked image to decompose it into corresponding sub bands and select LH2* and LL3* sub bands.
3. Extract watermark bits of Signature text watermark form LL3 sub band of cover image and LL3* sub band of watermarked image and Symptoms text watermark form LH2 sub band of cover image and LH2* sub band of watermarked image using equation

$$Wbt_i' = \frac{A_i'(x,y) - A_i(x,y)}{k^* A_i(x,y)}; i = \text{extracted symptoms } and \text{ signature watermark} \quad (8.11)$$

$A'(x,y)$ and $A(x,y)$ are DWT coefficients of cover and watermarked image respectively, Wbt_i' is extracted text watermarking bits and k is the gain factor.

4. Apply arithmetic decoding process to obtained watermark bits of symptoms watermark and convert watermark bits into text to obtain symptoms text watermark.
5. Apply Hamming decoder algorithm to obtained watermark bits of Signature watermark and convert watermark bits into text to obtain signature text watermark.

8.5   Experimental Results and Performance Analysis

The performance of the combined DWT-DCT-SVD watermarking algorithm has been evaluated in terms of quality of the watermarked image (PSNR), bit error rate (BER) of text watermarks and robustness of the watermarked image (NC) using BPNN. The gray-scale medical CT-scan image of size 512×512 as cover image, the Lump image of size 256×256 is considered as image watermark. For the healthcare applications security of the watermark has become an important factor. The security of the image watermark is enhanced by using Arnold transform is applied before embedding in to the cover. Signature and symptoms watermarks are considered as text watermark of size 190 characters. Signature watermark contains the doctor's signature/identification code and the symptoms watermark contains the patient diagnostic information. Robustness performance of the image watermark is improved by applying the Back Propagation Neural Network (BPNN). In order to reduce the BER performance of the proposed method, error correcting Hamming code (ECC) is applied to the ASCII representation of the signature watermark before embedding into the cover. In addition, lossless encoding method (arithmetic coding) is applied on the symptom watermark which can be correctly retrieving the diagnostic information of the patient. Strength of watermarks is varied by varying the gain factor in the proposed algorithm. For testing the robustness of the extracted watermarks (both image and text) and visual quality of watermarked cover medical image MATLAB is used. Figure 8.3a–c shows the cover CT-scan image, Lump image watermark and watermarked images respectively. Figure 8.4 shows the Signature and Symptoms text watermarks.

Figure 8.5a, b shows the extracted watermarks with and without using the BPNN training respectively. The PSNR, BER and NC performance of the proposed method is shown in Tables 8.2, 8.3, 8.4, 8.5, 8.6. In Table 8.2, the PSNR and

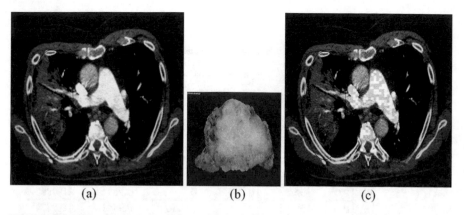

(a)   (b)   (c)

Fig. 8.3 (a) CTscan cover image (b) lump image watermark (c) watermarked image

Doctor's Signature/ID: BXBPS4999S1
Diagnostic Information
Hospital Code: JUITWAKNAGHAT
Patient No: 200_Ward_ABC
Symptoms: c/c Lump in right barest_No fever history_Pain in right shoulder_No history of retraction and discharge
from Hospital_Other reports_MammographNo 1568_FNAC39_B+_SOLAN

Fig. 8.4 Signature and Symptoms text watermarks

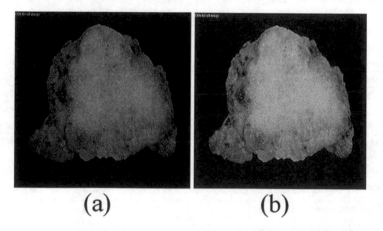

(a)   (b)

Fig. 8.5 Extracted Lump watermark (a) without and (b) with BPNN training

Table 8.2 PSNR, NC and BER performance of the proposed method at different gain

SN	Gain factor	PSNR (dB)	BER (Text Watermark)		NC values	
			Signature	Symptoms	Without BPNN	With BPNN
1	0.01	43.88	0	0.2174	0.9344	0.9547
2	0.02	41.22	0	0.1087	0.9764	0.9844
3	0.05	36.53	0	0	0.9846	0.9889
4	0.08	33.59	0	0	0.9861	0.9888
5	0.1	32.09	0	0	0.9852	0.9875
6	0.12	30.85	0	0	0.9853	0.9872
7	0.15	29.33	0	0	0.9849	0.9864
8	0.2	27.29	0	0	0.9851	0.9866

Table 8.3 PSNR, NC and BER performance for different no of characters in Symptoms watermark at different gain

SN	Number of characters	Gain factor	PSNR (dB)	BER		NC	
				Signature	Symptoms	Without BPNN	With BPNN
1	50	0.01	43.95	0	0.4202	0.9363	0.9563
		0.05	36.54	0	0	0.9846	0.9889
		0.1	32.12	0	0.4202	0.9853	0.9875
2	100	0.01	43.93	0	0.2110	0.9378	0.9573
		0.05	36.52	0	0	0.9846	0.9888
		0.1	32.10	0	0.2110	0.9851	0.9874
3	150	0.01	43.92	0	0	0.9356	0.9556
		0.05	36.51	0	0	0.9845	0.9887
		0.1	32.11	0	0	0.9854	0.9877
4	200	0.01	43.89	0	0.1370	0.9339	0.9541
		0.05	36.52	0	0	0.9847	0.9888
		0.1	32.09	0	0	0.9853	0.9877

Table 8.4 PSNR, NC and BER performance for different cover images at gain = 0.08

SN	Cover image	PSNR (dB)	BER (Text Watermark)		NC	
			Signature	Symptoms	Without BPNN	With BPNN
1	Brain	33.55	0	0	0.9745	0.9825
2	Mammography	32.94	0	0.1087	0.9474	0.9638
3	Ultrasound	34.34	0	0.4348	0.9642	0.9770
4	Lena	32.93	0	0	0.9795	0.9855
5	MRI	34.33	0	0	0.9869	0.9888
6	Mandrill	31.54	0	0	0.9845	0.9849

Table 8.5 PSNR and NC and BER performance for different text watermark size at gain 0.08

SN	Text watermark size (in characters)		PSNR (dB)	BER		NC	
	Signature	Symptoms		Signature	Symptoms	With BPNN	Without BPNN
1	12	10	33.62	0	0	0.9860	0.9886
2	12	20	33.62	0	0	0.9861	0.9887
3	12	50	33.60	0	0	0.9860	0.9887
4	12	75	33.60	0	0	0.9862	0.9888
5	12	100	33.59	0	0	0.9861	0.9889
6	12	150	33.61	0	0	0.9861	0.9886
7	12	200	33.61	0	0	0.9861	0.9887

Table 8.6 BER and NC performance of the proposed method for different attacks at gain = 0.08

SN	Attacks	BER		NC	
		Signature	Symptoms	With BPNN	Without BPNN
1	JPEG 10	0	0.1087	0.2081	0.3120
2	JPEG 30	0	0	0.9733	0.9803
3	JPEG 60	0	0	0.9679	0.9703
4	JPEG 80	0	0	0.9812	0.9871
5	JPEG 100	0	0	0.9860	0.9886
6	Salt & Peppers (density = 0.02)	0	0.2031	0.6926	0.7013
7	Salt & Peppers (density = 0.01)	0	0	0.7569	0.7747
8	Salt & Peppers (density = 0.001)	0	0	0.9604	0.9658
9	Gaussian(Mean = 0.01,Variance = 0.002)	0	0.2174	0.8365	0.8748
10	Gaussian (Mean = 0, Variance = 0.001)	0	0	0.9307	0.9466
11	Gaussian (Mean = 0.01,Variance = 0.0005)	0	0	0.9741	0.9761
12	Average filtering	0	0.1087	0.9824	0.9869
13	Low pass filtering	0	0.1087	0.9852	0.9889
14	Median filtering	0	0.2237	0.0025	0.0123
15	Speckle (Variance = 0.02)	0.1119	28.57	0.8286	0.8673
16	Speckle (Variance = 0.01)	0.1119	10.7143	0.9024	0.9286
17	Speckle (Variance = 0.005)	0	0	0.9860	0.9886
18	Rotation (2°)	0.3356	2.3810	0.4022	0.4442
19	Crop (6.25%)	0.4474	47.619	0.8691	0.9059
20	Resize (512-410-512)	0	0.3356	0.9177	0.9377
21	JPEG80 + Gaussian(M = 0.01,V = 0.002)	0	0.1119	0.8135	0.8558
22	JPEG80 + Salt & Peppers (d = 0.002)	0	0	0.9074	0.9312
23	Gaussian(M = 0.01,V = 0.002) + Speckle (V = 0.005)	0	0.2237	0.7901	0.8276
24	Salt & Peppers(d = 0.002) + Speckle (V = 0.005)	0.2237	1.1905	0.7947	0.8328
25	JPEG80 + Speckle (V = 0.005)	0	0.2237	0.9585	0.9645

NC performance of the proposed method has been evaluated without any noise attack. Without using the BPNN, the maximum PSNR value is 43.88 dB and NC value is 0.9344 at gain factor = 0.01. However, the NC value is obtained as 0.9547 with BPNN at the same gain. With BPNN, the maximum NC value is obtained as 0.9888 at gain factor = 0.08. However, the NC value has been obtained as 0.9861 without using the BPNN at same gain factor.

The BER value for signature watermark is '0' at all considered gain factors. However, BER value of the Symptoms watermark is 0.2174 and 0.1087 for gain factors 0.01 and 0.02 respectively. Referring Table 8.2, we found that larger the gain factor, stronger the robustness and smaller the gain factor, better the visual

PSNR, NC and BER performance of the proposed method at different gain

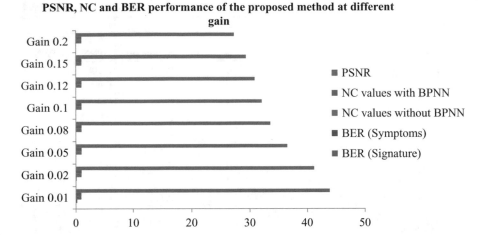

Fig. 8.6 PSNR, NC and BER performance of the proposed method at different gain factor

quality of the watermarked image. The graphical representation of Table 8.2 is shown in Fig. 8.6.

The gain factor '0.08' is considered for the experimental purpose in Tables 8.3, 8.4, 8.5, 8.6. Table 8.3 shows the PSNR, BER and NC (with and without using BPNN) performance of the proposed method for different size of text watermarks. The maximum PSNR value is obtained at gain factor 0.01, which is 43.95 dB. However, the NC value obtained is 0.9363 (without using BPNN) for 50 characters of Symptoms watermark at the same gain factor. Refereeing this table, the maximum NC value is 0.9889 (with BPNN) at gain factor 0.05 for 50 characters of Symptoms watermark. The BER value of the signature watermark is '0' at all chosen gain factors. However, the BER value is 0.4202 for the Symptoms watermark at gain = 0.01. The maximum BER value is 0.4202, which can be recovered all the bits at higher gain value.

Table 8.4 shows the PSNR, BER and NC (with and without using BPNN) performance of the proposed method for six different cover images. With BPNN, the highest NC values (0.9888) have been obtained with MRI image at gain = 0.08 for Lump image. However the minimum NC value is 0.9638 for Mammography image at the same gain. Referencing this Table, the highest BER value has been obtained for Ultrasound image, which is 0.4348. However, the minimum BER value is '0' for all other cover images except the Mammography and Ultrasound images. Figure 8.7 shows the graphical representation of Table 8.4. Table 8.5 shows the PSNR, BER and NC performance of proposed algorithm for different size of the symptoms watermark. In this table, the size of the Signature watermark is fixed and the size of Symptoms watermark is varied. Referring this table, the BER value is found to be '0' for all different size of the symptoms watermark. Figure 8.8 show the graphical representation of Table 8.5. Table 8.6 shows the BER and NC performance of the proposed method for different attacks [11].

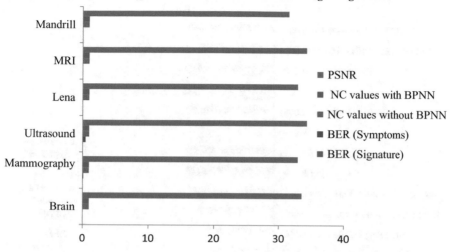

Fig. 8.7 PSNR, NC and BER performance of the proposed method for different cover image

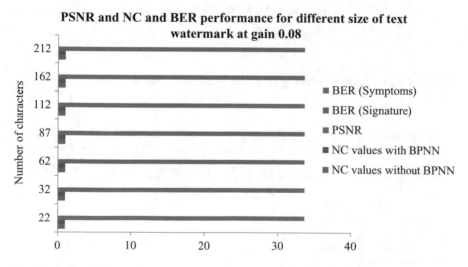

Fig. 8.8 PSNR, NC and BER performance of the proposed method for different size of text watermark

Without BPNN, the highest NC value has been obtained as 0.9852 for Gaussian low pass filtering. However, the lowest NC is 0.0025 for JPEG (QF = 10) attack. With BPNN, the highest NC value has been obtained as 0.9889 for Gaussian low pass filtering. However, the lowest NC is 0.0123 for Median filtering attack. Refereeing this table, the highest BER of Symptoms and Signature watermark is

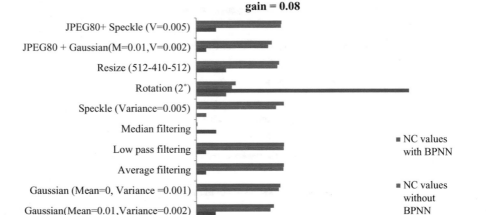

Fig. 8.9 NC and BER performance of the proposed method for known attacks

Table 8.7 Comparison results under NC value

SN	Attacks	Singh et al. [12]	Ganic et al. [28]	Proposed method
1.	JPEG 30	–	0.141	0.9787
2.	Resize (512-256-512)	–	−0.211	0.7902
3.	Gaussian noise (Mean = 0, variance = 0.3)	–	0.271	0.6583
4.	Gaussian noise (Mean = 0, variance = 0.5)	0.6565	–	0.6576
5.	Gaussian noise (Mean = 0, variance = 0.001)	0.9365	–	0.9466
6.	Salt & Peppers (density = 0.5)	0.6069	–	0.6587
7.	Salt & Peppers (density = 0.5)	0.7552	–	0.7747
8.	Gaussian LPF (Standard Deviation = 0.6)	0.9343	–	0.9883
9.	Histogram Equilization	0.569	0.716	0.9404

Table 8.8 Subjective measure of the watermarked image quality at different gain factor

Gain factors	Quality of the watermarked image
0.01	Excellent visual quality of the watermarked image
0.05	Very good visual quality of the watermarked image
0.1	Good visual quality of the watermarked image
0.15	Average/acceptable visual quality of the watermarked image
0.2	Poor visual quality of the watermarked image
0.5	Very poor visual quality of the watermarked image

47.619% and 0.4474% for Crop attack respectively. However, the minimum BER value is '0'. Figure 8.9 show the graphical representation of Table 8.6.

Table 8.7 show the NC performance of the proposed method is compared with other reported techniques [12, 28]. The maximum NC value obtained by the Singh et al. [12] and Ganic et al. [28] is 0.9365 and 0.716 respectively. However, the maximum NC value obtained by the proposed method is 0.9883. Referring Table 8.7 it is established that the proposed method obtained NC value range from 0.6576 to 0.9883. However, NC value range as obtained by the Singh et al. from 0.569 to 0.9365 and Ganic et al. from −0.211 to 0.716. The proposed method offer higher robustness than the other two reported techniques. Finally, the quality of the watermarked image is evaluated by the subjective technique also [12] in Table 8.8. Six different persons are involved who have to vote for the quality of a medium in a controlled test environment. This can be done by simply providing a distorted medium of which the quality has to be evaluated by the subject. Referring Table 8.8 it is established that the quality of the watermarked images is acceptable for diagnosis at all the chosen gain factors except the gain factor = 0.2 and 0.5, which shows the poor/very poor visual quality of the watermarked image. Based on the above discussion, the proposed method highly depends on the gain factors, size if the image and text watermark and different noise variations.

8.6   Summary

In this chapter, a novel method for multiple watermarking based on DWT, DCT and SVD has been presented using Back Propagation Neural Network. The suggested method considered gray scale images for the experimental purpose. However, the watermark embedding into color image provides greater space against the watermark embedding into gray scale image. The performance of the watermarking system will greatly depends on the choice of color space and selection of embedding color channel. The main properties of the proposed work is identified as follows:

1. The fusion of DWT, DCT and SVD offer better performance in terms of imperceptibility, robustness and capacity as compared to DWT, DCT and SVD applied individually.
2. Embedding more than one watermark within the cover image reduces the storage capacity and the bandwidth requirements. The storage and bandwidth requirements are very important in medical applications.
3. For enhancing the robustness of the image watermark, BPNN is applied to the extracted watermark which gives the higher NC values compared to without using the BPNN.
4. Security and confidentiality are provided by scrambling the Lump watermark using Arnold transforms before embedding into the cover.
5. Lossless arithmetic compression is applieded to Symptoms watermark before embedding in to the cover for the bit compactness. The lossless compression techniques is also preffered in medical applications in which every bit information is preserved before and after the compression process.
6. To increase the robustness of the signature watermark and reduce the channel distortion, Hamming error correcting code is applied to the watermark before embedding into the cover, and
7. Finally, the visual quality of the watermarked image is evaluated by the subjective method also. Therefore, proposed method provides a valuable solution for the prevention of patient identity theft in healthcare applications such as tele-ophthalmology, tele-medicine, tele-diagnosis and tele-consultancy etc.

In future, the performance of the suggested wavelet based image watermarking method can be extended for their application to video watermarking.

References

1. H. Nyeem, W. Boles, C. Boyd, A review of medical image watermarking requirements for teleradiology. J. Digit. Imaging **26**(2), 326–343 (2013)
2. A.M. Elmisery, S. Rho, D. Botvich, A distributed collaborative platform for personal health profiles in patient-driven health social network. IJDSN Hindawi Publ. Corp. **2015**, 1–12 (2015)
3. A.K. Singh, B. Kumar, M. Dave, A. Mohan, Multiple watermarking on medical images using selective DWT coefficients. J. Med. Imaging Health Inf. **5**(3), 607–614 (2015)
4. A.K. Singh, M. Dave, A. Mohan, Robust and secure multiple watermarking in wavelet domain. A special issue on advanced signal processing technologies and systems for healthcare applications (ASPTSHA). J. Med. Imaging Health Inf. **5**(2), 406–414 (2015)
5. A. Giakoumaki, S. Pavlopoulos, D. Koutsouris, Secure and efficient health data management through multiple watermarking on medical images. Med. Biol. Eng. Comput. **44**, 619–631 (2006)
6. A. Giakoumaki, S. Pavlopoulos, D. Koutsouris, Multiple image watermarking applied to health information management. IEEE Trans. Inf. Technol. Biomed. **10**, 722–732 (2006)
7. A.K. Singh, Improved hybrid technique for robust and imperceptible multiple watermarking using digital images. Multimedia Tools Appl. **76**(6), 8881–8900 (2017)
8. M. Terry, Medical identity theft and telemedicine security. Telemed. e-Health **15**(10), 928–932 (2009)

9. D. Bowman, http://www.fiercehealthit.com/story/researchers-use-digital-watermarks-protect-medical-images (2012)
10. M. Ollove, www.usatoday.com/story/.../stateline-identity-thefts-medical.../5279351 (2014)
11. A.K. Singh, B. Kumar, M. Dave, S.P. Ghrera, A. Mohan, Digital image watermarking: techniques and emerging applications, in *Handbook of Research on Modern Cryptographic Solutions for Computer and Cyber Security* (IGI Global, Hershey, 2016), pp. 246–272
12. A.K. Singh, M. Dave, A. Mohan, Hybrid technique for robust and imperceptible multiple watermarking using medical images. J. Multimedia Tools Appl. **75**(14), 8381–8401 (2016)
13. A. Kannammal, S. Subha Rani, Two level security for medical images using watermarking/encryption algorithms. Int. J. Imaging Syst. Technol. **24**(1), 111–120 (2014)
14. K. Pal, G. Ghosh, M. Bhattacharya, Biomedical image watermarking in wavelet domain for data integrity using bit majority algorithm and multiple copies of hidden information. Am. J. Biomed. Eng. **2**(2), 29–37 (2012)
15. A.K. Singh, M. Dave, A. Mohan, Multilevel encrypted text watermarking on medical images using spread-spectrum in DWT domain. Wireless Personal Commun.: Int. J. **83**(3), 2133–2150 (2015)
16. B. Kumar, H.V. Singh, S.P. Singh, A. Mohan, Secure spread-spectrum watermarking for telemedicine applications. J. Inf. Secur. **2**, 91–98 (2011)
17. B. Kumar, A. Anand, S.P. Singh, A. Mohan, High capacity spread-spectrum watermarking for telemedicine applications. World Acad. Sci. Eng. Technol. **5**, 62–66 (2011)
18. I.J. Cox, J. Kilian, L.F. Thomson, S. Talal, Secure spread spectrum watermarking for multimedia. IEEE Trans. Image Process. **6**(12), 1673–1687 (1997)
19. A.K. Singh, B. Kumar, M. Dave, A. Mohan, Robust and imperceptible spread-spectrum watermarking for telemedicine applications. Proc. Natl. Acad. Sci., India, Sect. A: Phys. Sci. **85**(2), 295–301 (2015)
20. A. Sharma, A.K. Singh, S.P. Ghrera, Robust and secure multiple watermarking technique for medical images. Wirel. Pers. Commun. **92**(4), 1611–1624 (2017)
21. R. Pandey, A.K. Singh, B. Kumar, A. Mohan, Iris based secure NROI multiple eye image watermarking for teleophthalmology. Multimedia Tools Appl. **75**(22), 14381–14397 (2016)
22. Z. Wei, H. Li, J. Dai, S. Wang, Image watermarking based on genetic algorithm, in IEEE International Conference on Multimedia and Expo, Toronto, ON, pp. 1117–1120, 2006
23. V. Aslantas, A.L. Dogan, S. Ozturk, DWT-SVD based image watermarking using particle swarm optimizer, in IEEE International Conference on Multimedia and Expo, Hannover, pp. 241–244, 2008
24. V. Aslantas, S. Ozer, S. Ozturk, Improving the performance of DCT-based fragile watermarking using intelligent optimization algorithms. Opt. Commun. **282**(14), 2806–2817 (2009)
25. V. Aslantas, An optimal robust digital image watermarking based on SVD using differential evolution algorithm. Opt. Commun. **282**(5), 769–777 (2009)
26. A.R.N. Nilchi, A. Taheri, A new robust digital image watermarking technique based on the discrete cosine transformation and neural network, in International Symposium on Biometrics and Security Technologies, Islamabad, pp. 1–7, 2008
27. C.T. Yen, Y.J. Huang, Frequency domain digital watermark recognition using image code sequences with a back-propagation neural network, Multimedia Tools Appl. **75**(16), 9745–9755 (2016)
28. E. Ganic, A.M. Eskicioglu, Robust DWT-SVD domain image watermarking: embedding data in all frequencies, in Proceedings of the 2004 Workshop on Multimedia and Security, ACM, pp. 166–174, 2004
29. N. Terzjia, M. Repges, K. Luck, W. Geisselhardt, Digital image watermarking using discrete wavelet transform: performance comparison of error correction codes, in International Association of Science and Technology for Development, 2002
30. C.-C. Lai, C.-C. Tsai, Digital image watermarking using discrete wavelet transform and singular value decomposition. IEEE Trans. Instrum. Meas. **59**(11), 3060–3063 (2010)

31. M. Vafaei, H. Mahdavi-Nasab, H. Pourghassem, A new robust blind watermarking method based on neural networks in wavelet transform domain. World Appl. Sci. J. **22**(11), 1572–1580 (2013)

32. M. Ali, C. WookAhn, P. Siarry, Differential evolution algorithm for the selection of optimal scaling factors in image watermarking. Special issue on advances in evolutionary optimization based image processing. Eng. Appl. Artif. Intell. **31**, 15–26 (2014)

33. A. Mehto, N. Mehra, Adaptive lossless medical image watermarking algorithm based on DCT & DWT. Proc. Computer Sci. **78**, 88–94 (2016)

34. T.S. Nguyen, C.C. Chang, X.Q. Yang, A reversible image authentication scheme based on fragile watermarking in discrete wavelet transform domain. AEU-Int. J. Electron. Commun. **70**(8), 1055–1061 (2016)

35. M. Shi-chun, L. Ren-hou, D. Hong-mei, W. Yun-kuan, Decision of image watermarking strength based on artificial neural-networks, in Proceedings of the 9th International Conference on Neural Information Processing, pp. 2430–2434, 2002

36. Y. Qun-ting, G. Tie-gang, L. Fan, A novel robust watermarking scheme based on neural network, in International Conference on Intelligent Computing and Integrated Systems (ICISS), IEEE, pp. 71–75, 2010

37. N. Mohananthini, G. Yamuna, Watermarking for images using wavelet domain in Back-Propagation neural network, in Advances in Engineering, Science and Management, pp. 100–105, 2012

38. M. Barni, F. Bartolini, Improved wavelet-based watermarking through pixel-wise masking. IEEE Trans. Image Process. **10**(5), 783–791 (2001)

39. A. Zear, A.K. Singh, P. Kumar, Multiple watermarking for healthcare applications. J. Intell. Syst. (2016). doi: 10.1515/jisys-2016-0036

40. B. Zeng, Reduction of blocking effect in DCT-coded images using zero-masking techniques. Signal Process. **79**(2), 205–211 (1999)

41. J.-M. Guo, H. Prasetyo, False-positive-free SVD-based image watermarking. J. Vis. Commun. Image Represent. **25**(5), 1149–1163 (2014)

42. F.N. Thakkar, V.K. Srivastava, A blind medical image watermarking: DWT-SVD based robust and secure approach for telemedicine applications. Multimedia Tools Appl. **76**(3), 3669–3697 (2017)

43. M. Cilimkovic, Neural networks and back propagation algorithm, Master Thesis, Institute of Technology, Ireland, 2013

Chapter 9
Securing Patient Data Through Multiple Watermarking and Selective Encryption

Amit Kumar Singh, Basant Kumar, Ghanshyam Singh, and Anand Mohan

9.1 Introduction

In recent year, every second a lot of multimedia documents/contents such as images, text, audio and video are created and transmitted all around the world through different social network/open channel different portals, websites and various applications [1]. The multimedia documents distribution over online social network/open channel using information and communication Technology (ICT) has proved an indispensible and cost effective technique for dissemination of the multimedia documents [2]. However, prevention of copyright violation, authenticity, confidentiality and ownership identity theft have been potential issues due attempts of malicious attacks/hacking of transmitted information on online social network/open channel [2–5]. It includes criminal offence ranging from ownership identity theft to

A.K. Singh (✉)
Department of Computer Science & Engineering, Jaypee University
of Information Technology, Waknaghat, Solan, India
e-mail: amit_245singh@yahoo.com

B. Kumar
Department of Electronics and Communication Engineering, Motilal Nehru
National Institute of Technology, Allahabad, India
e-mail: singhbasant@yahoo.com

G. Singh
Department of Electronics and Communication Engineering, Jaypee University
of Information Technology, Waknaghat, Solan, India
e-mail: drghanshyam.singh@yahoo.com

A. Mohan
Department of Electronics Engineering, Indian Institute of Technology (BHU),
Varanasi, India
e-mail: profanandmohan@gmail.com

© Springer International Publishing AG 2017
A.K. Singh et al. (eds.), *Medical Image Watermarking*, Multimedia Systems
and Applications, DOI 10.1007/978-3-319-57699-2_9

copyright violation and from personal information exposure to medical history disclosure is being made every day [5]. In general, some watermark information is embedding into digital/multimedia documents to ensure the authenticity of digital/multimedia documents as required in several important applications [1, 2, 4–8]. It includes e-health, fingerprinting, forensic, protection of social digital contents, E-Voting, driver licenses, military, remote education, media file archiving, broadcast monitoring and digital cinema.

Therefore, the researcher are required to propose robust and secure watermarking techniques for illegal access or alteration of such multimedia documents transmitted or uploaded over unsecured channels. Further, various researcher/scientist strive to develop different watermarking techniques for improving one or a subset of benchmark parameters. The major benchmark parameters of the digital watermark are imperceptibility, robustness, security, data pay load and computational complexity, which have been discussed detail in [2]. However, it is clear that they compromise with other remaining parameters. Thus, there is need to develop effective watermarking methods that can offer good trade-off between these benchmark parameters for the above considered applications. The proposed research/work focuses on to optimize trade-off between these benchmark parameters.

For the above extensive discussion, the secure transmission of multimedia/social/e-health contents on online social unsecured networks as well as its related security concerns, the present research focuses on image watermarking to ensure guaranteed authenticity of transmitted multimedia information. The image watermarking is a value added/security tool for hiding digital information into multimedia documents. The hidden watermark can be later extracted or detected for the purpose of multimedia document security. The significant importance of the image watermarking are minimize the storage space and bandwidth requirements, privacy of the personal data, and protection against tampering [1, 4, 5, 9]. Presently, the cryptography, stegnography and watermarking are three popular techniques for multimedia document security [2]. The fundamental differences between these three concepts are presented in Table 9.1.

Table 9.1 Important difference between cryptography, stegnography and watermarking

Cryptography	Stegnography	Watermarking
Secret writing	Covered writing	Covered writing
Protecting the content	Concealing the message while focus on the bandwidth of the hidden message	Hide the message and robustness is the key performance parameter against attacks
Sending massage in different form	Just hide the any message in multimedia objects	It always hide the information of a digital object
Require secret transmission	Secret transmission is not required	Secret transmission is not required
Massage will unsecure once the it is decrypted, which is required for human perception	Hide the message within cover, no one can detect it	Hide the message and message remains in the cover after decryption

The image watermarking techniques can categorized into spatial and transform domain techniques [10]. The transform domain techniques are more complex and robust than the spatial domain techniques, as reported by various surveys [2, 11–14].

The subsequent section of the chapter is structured as follows: The related and recent state-of-the-art techniques are provided in Sec. 9.2. The main contribution of the work is summarized in Sect. 9.3. Section 9.4 describes the proposed multiple watermarking framework. Experimental results and brief analysis of the work is reported in Sect.9.5. Next, summary of chapter is presented in Sect. 9.6.

9.2   Related Work

In this section, a brief review of related and recent transform domain based image watermarking methods is presented below:

Kannammal and Subha Rani [15] proposed a encryption based secure medical image watermarking method using DWT and LSB. The method is applied well known encryption techniques AES, RSA and RC4 on watermarked image in which RC4 encryption technique offer good performance than other two encryption techniques. In addition, the method is robust for different signal processing attacks. Al-Haj and Amer [16] presented robust watermarking method based on LSB, DWT and SVD. In the embedding of two different watermarks, the robust watermark is embedded in region-of-non-interest (RONI) part of the host image using DWT and SVD and the fragile watermarks is embedded into region-of-interest (ROI) part of the image by using the LSB method. The proposed method offers high robustness for JPEG and salt & pepper attacks. Xing and Tan [17] proposed a color image watermarking based on SVD, log polarmap-ping (LPM) and phase correlation methods. The experimental results shown that the method is robust for Gaussian noise addition, lossy JPEG compression, low pass filtering, and waveform attacks. In addition, the robustness is improved for geometrical attacks by evaluating the phase correlation in image LPM domain before embedding the watermark into the cover. Ghafoor and Imran [18] proposed a non-blind color image watermarking method using principle component analysis (PCA), discrete wavelet transform and singular value decomposition. The method is imperceptible and robust for different kinds of signal processing attacks. In addition, the PSNR performance of the method is compared and found to be the visual quality of the method is better than other reported techniques. Santhi and Thangavelu [19] presents a method for color image watermarking using DWT, DCT and SVD. For improving the robustness of the watermark, the most significant coefficients are selected for the embedding of the watermark. The robustness of the extracted watermark is tested for different known attacks and found to be the method is robust except for rotation attacks. A secure and robust watermarking method based DWT and DCT is presented by Zhao and Dang [20]. The method is robust for known attacks. In addition, the security of the watermark is enhanced by using logistic chaotic encryption to encrypt the mark.

Xiong [21] presents a method for color image watermarking based on 3D-DCT. In the embedding process, RGB color image is divided into non-overlapping blocks and then 3D-DCT transform is applied on each block to embed a bit watermarking into each block's using quantization method. The method is imperceptible and robust for different known attacks. The visual quality of watermarked image and the robustness of the extracted watermark is compared with other reported techniques.

Shi et al. [22] present a color image watermark embedding technique based on SVD. The robustness of the watermark is enhanced by using the image scrambling and blocked with circulation. The authors reported that the experimental result of the proposed method is highly imperceptible and robust for different known attacks. Ramamurthy and Varadarajan [23] proposed a blind color image watermarking method to embed bitmap is considered as watermark. For improving the robustness of the watermark, BPNN is applied on the extracted watermark to reduce the noise/ distortion effect on the watermarked image. Experimental results show that the method is robust for different attacks. The authors claimed that the visual quality of the method is better than that of the other reported techniques [24]. A region based robust and secure watermarking method through DWT and DCT for medical applications is presented by Sharma et al. [25]. For improving the security of the considered image and text watermark are first encoded by message-digest (MD5) hash algorithm and Rivest–Shamir–Adleman (RSA), respectively, and then both the encoded watermark is embedding into the medical cover image. In order to enhance the robustness of the text watermark Hamming error correction code is also applied on the encrypted watermark. The method is robust for selected known attacks. Zear et al. [26] proposed a robust and secure multiple watermarking technique through DWT, DCT, SVD and neural network. Two different text watermark information is compressed and encoded by arithmetic and Hamming error correction code respectively. The compressed and encoded text watermark is embedding into the cover medical image. Further, Arnold transform is applied on the image watermark before embedding into the cover. The performance of the algorithm has been extensively evaluated in terms of PSNR, NC and BER. Pandey et al. [27] presents a secure DWT and SVD based multiple watermarking methods for tele-ophthalmology applications. The method embeds multiple watermarks in the non-region of interest (NROI) region of the DWT cover image. The method is robust for signal processing and "Checkmark" attacks. Mary et al. [28] proposed a encryption and compression based watermarking method in LSB domain. The cover and watermark image is compressed and encrypted by JPEG 2000 compression technique and modified RC6 block cipher respectively before the embedding process. Further, the encrypted watermark image is embedding into the compressed cover image using LSB to addressing the robustness, capacity and security of the watermarking system. A lossless compression based watermarking technique is proposed by Badshah et al. [29] using teleradiology images. The ROI part of the watermark is considered along with a key to generate a new watermark. The generated watermark is compressed by Lempel–Ziv–Welch(LZW) technique and the compressed watermark is embedding into the RONI part of the cover image. The experimental results established that the performance of the different compression method is investigated and found that the LZW compression technique offer better compression ratio performance than other conventional compression techniques. The method also verifies the tempering in the watermark after extraction and decompression process.

9.3   Important Contribution of the Work

The proposed multiple watermarking method based on DWT, DCT, SVD, BPNN, error correcting codes (Hamming and BCH) and selective encryption. The major advantages of wavelet based watermarking are space frequency localization, multi-resolution representation, multi-scale analysis, adaptability, linear complexity and support JPEG 2000 image standard [2]. However, the important limitations of DWT are shift sensitive, poor directionality and shortage of phase information [26]. Further, the watermark information based on its importance can be embedded at higher level DWT sub-bands [2], which is an essential requirement for data management in various applications. Due to good energy compaction property of the DCT and SVD, it enhances the robustness and imperceptibility performance of the watermarking systems [9]. The DCT has been applied on the DWT coefficient to presents the important information in very small number of low frequency components. However, major drawback of DCT and SVD is blocking artifact and computationally expensive respectively [26]. The false positive problem is another drawback of the SVD based watermarking techniques [30, 31]. This problem is easily solved by the method proposed in [30] and [31]. Various researchers have been reported that the watermarking technique using DWT, DCT and SVD. It is observed that the robustness performance of the hybrid technique (DWT, DCT and SVD) is better than the technique using DWT, DCT or SVD individually [2, 9, 26].

In this chapter, due to higher data embedding capacity of image, the present work focuses on watermarking technique using image as cover/host media. The proposed multiple watermarking method is embedding two watermarks in the form of image and text simultaneously. This simultaneously watermark embedding method has fewer constraints than the other two dual watermarks methods [32–34]. In addition, the simultaneously embedding method can easily make two watermarks non-interfering with a proper division, thus provides an effective way to guarantee the quality of the two watermarks. Table 9.2 shows the summary of considered techniques in the proposed method and objectives achieved by using these techniques. The main contribution of the work is summarized as follows:

1. *Capacity of embedding multiple watermarks*: The method proposed in [18–23, 35–44] has been embedded only single watermark either in the form of image or text. However, the proposed method can embed multiple watermarks (text and image both) simultaneously, which enhance the security of multimedia documents with the acceptable performance of robustness and imperceptibility. The other advantages of multiple watermarking over the single watermarking for the important applications such as medical [45] as well as social applications are given in Table 9.2. To address the issue of ownership identity authentication, multiple watermarks have been embedded into the same multimedia objects simultaneously.

Table 9.2 Summary of considered techniques and corresponding objectives

Using techniques	Objectives achieved by using the techniques
Multiple watermarks/documents	The watermarking techniques using single watermark is unsuitable for some practical applications. However, multiple watermarks instead of single are the various advantages such as – enhances robustness and security of the hidden watermark – reduced storage and bandwidth requirements during transmission, and – prevention form tempering and identity theft, and – the hidden watermark can be acting as keywords for efficient archiving and data retrieval for queering mechanism However, multiple watermarking increases the computational complexity and reduces the quality of the watermarked image
Transform domain techniques such as DWT, DCT and SVD	More robust than the spatial domain techniques
BPNN	Improve the robustness of image watermark/document
BCH and Hamming ECCs	Improve robustness of the personal information watermark or reduce BER values for received watermarks bit information
Selective encryption	Enhance Security of the watermarked image i.e. cover, image and text watermarks
Health data management	Address the health/personal data management issues by embedding the more robust data at higher level DWT sub-band and less robust data at lower level DWT sub-band

This simultaneous multiple watermarking technique is better than the other two multiple watermarks embedding methods reported in [30–32].

2. *Improved performance*: Tables 9.4, 9.5, 9.6, 9.7, 9.8, 9.9 show the NC performance of the proposed method is enhanced by using BPNN training. Refereeing these tables it is established that the BER performance of the proposed method is investigated by two important error correcting code (Hamming and BCH). It is found that the BCH code offer better performance (ability to corrects more error) than Hamming code. In Tables 9.11 and 9.12, the method is compared with other reported techniques and has been found to be giving superior performance for robustness as suggested by the method reported in [18–22].

3. *Enhance the security*: Security of the host and watermarks is enhanced by using selective encryption technique. In recent year, the selective encryption is a new approach to reduce the computational requirements for large size of multimedia contents/documents to offers confidentiality in secure multimedia contents on online social network/e-health/real time applications as well as many other applications [46]. In this encryption technique, only important parts/any one of the color channels of the cover media contents is encrypted. The encryption may

also provide a potential solution to existing problem of patient identity theft and guaranteed authenticity of transmitted information in e-health applications as well as other applications of secure document dissemination.

4. *Reduced storage and bandwidth requirements*: The multimedia cover files in form of medical image contain important information in the form of image and text. Further, in order to conserve the transmission bandwidth requirement or storage space minimization the personal details may be embedded inside the cover image [2].

5. *Robust data management*: The proposed multiple watermarking methods attempted to simultaneously address the health data management issues such as data security, data compaction, unauthorized access and temper proofing, having different characteristics and requirements [2].

9.4   The Proposed Framework

The proposed method is based on DWT, DCT, SVD, ECC, BPNN and selective encryption, which enhance the robustness and security without significant degradation of the image quality for different signal processing attacks. The proposed technique initially decomposes the host image into third level DWT. To addressing the data management issue as given in Table 9.3, the higher robust data (personal information/text watermark) and less robust data (image watermark) are embedding into the low frequency band (LL3) at the third level and vertical frequency band (LH2) at second level DWT, respectively.

The robustness of image watermark is enhanced by using Back Propagation Neural Network (BPNN) is applied to the extracted watermark. In order to reduce the BER performance of the proposed method, two different ECCs (Hamming and BCH) is applied on personal information data before embedding into the host image. Further, the BER performance of Hamming and BCH ECCs on the text

Table 9.3 Allocation of watermarks according to robustness and capacity criteria at different DWT sub-band

Sub-band used	Embedded watermark			Description of the considered watermarks
	Watermark types	Robustness requirements	Watermark size (bits)	
LH2	Image	High	128×128	Image watermark. To check the robustness against attacks and the purpose of data integrity control
LL3	Personal information	Very high	100 characters	Text watermark. It contains the doctor's identification code, keywords and patient's personal and examination data. The doctor's identification code used for origin authentication, index for each type of disease and reduce the storage and bandwidth requirement

watermark considered as personal information has been investigated. Figure 9.1a, b shows the image and text watermarks embedding and extraction process respectively. Figure 9.2 show the BPNN training process. The proposed algorithm has three major parts as given below subsections.

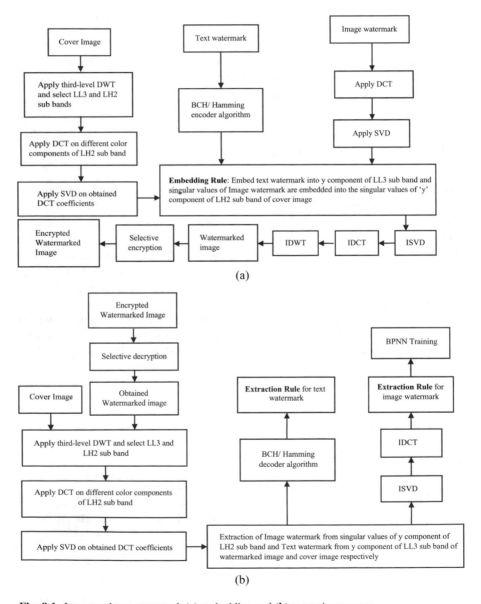

Fig. 9.1 Image and text watermark (**a**) embedding and (**b**) extraction process

Fig. 9.2 BPNN Training
Process for image
watermark [26]

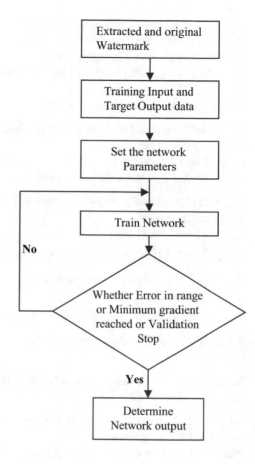

9.4.1   Algorithm 1: Image Watermark Embedding
and Extraction Process

The detail of the embedding and extraction algorithms are discuss below:

start:
STEP 1: Initialization and inputs

STEP 2: Read the Images
Host Image ← Kidney.jpg (Medical host image of size 512×512)
Watermark Image ← Stone.jpg (Watermark image of size 128×128)

**STEP 3: Determine DWT coefficients of the host and DCT coefficients of the
Watermark image**
//Apply first level DWT on host image
$[LL_1 , LH_1 , HL_1 , HH_1]$ ← DWT (Host, Haar wavelet);

//Apply second level DWT on host image
$[LL_2 , LH_2 , HL_2 , HH_2] \leftarrow$ DWT (LL_1, Haar wavelet);
//Apply third level DWT on host image
$[LL_3 , LH_3 , HL_3 , HH_3] \leftarrow$ DWT (LL_2, Haar wavelet);
//Apply DCT on watermark image
W_DCT $\leftarrow$ DCT(watermark_image);

STEP 4: Choice of LH_2 subands of the host cover and obtain the DCT coefficients for the same
if (DCT on LH_2) **then**
H_DCT$\leftarrow$ DCT (LH_2); Otherwise, **endif;**

STEP 5: Compute the singular values of DCT coefficients for medical host and Watermark image
if (SVD on H_DCT) **then**

$U_h S_h V_h^T \leftarrow SVD\left(H\_DCT\right)$; Otherwise, **endif;**

// $U_h and V_h^T$: orthonormal matrices and S_h are the singular values of the host image
if (SVD on W_DCT) **then**

$U_w S_w V_w^T \leftarrow SVD\left(W\_DCT\right)$; Otherwise, **endif;**

// $U_w and V_w^T$: orthonormal matrices and S_w are the singular values of the watermark image

STEP 6: Embed the image watermark in to host image
$S_h + kS_w = Host\_embed$; for gain (k) = 0.01 to 0.12.

Step 7: Find the Watermarked Image using inverse_SVD, inverse_DCT and inverse_DWT respectively
Watermarked_Img $\leftarrow$ (LL_2 , Host_embed , HL_2 , HH_2)**end;**

Step 8: Apply selective encryption on watermarked image (containing both image and text) and decryption on encrypted watermarked imag
Encrypted_Watermarked $\leftarrow$ Selective_encr (*Watermarked_Img*);
Decrypted_Watermarked $\leftarrow$ Selective_decr (Encrypted_Watermarked);
end;

Step 9: Determine DWT coefficients (sub-bands) of possibly distorted decrypted watermarked image
//Apply up to third level DWT on watermarked image
[w_LL1,w_LH1,w_HL1,w_HH1]=DWT(Decrypted_Watermarked, Haar wavelet);
[w_LL2,w_LH2,w_HL2,w_HH2]= DWT(w_LL1,Haar wavelet);
[w_LL3,w_LH3,w_HL3,w_HH3]=DWT(w_LL2, Haar wavelet);

Step 10: Compute the DCT coefficients of selected sub-band (w_LH2) of DWT
W1_DCT $\leftarrow$DCT(w_LH2);

STEP 11: Compute the singular values of DCT coefficients
if (SVD on W1_DCT) **then**

$U_{hw} S_{hw} V_{hw}^T \quad SVD(\text{W1}\_DCT)$; Otherwise, **endif;**

STEP 12: Extract the image watermark from the decrypted watermarked image

$S_{EW} \leftarrow (S_{hw}\text{-}S_h)/k$; for gain (k) = 0.01 to 0.12. **endif;**
//modified DWT coefficients
Watr $\quad U_w S_{EW} V_w^T$
Extracted_Watermark $\leftarrow$ inverse_DCT(Watr); **end;**

STEP 13: Apply back propagation neural network on extracted watermark

9.4.2 Algorithm 2: Text Watermark Embedding and Extraction Process

The text watermark is converted into a bit stream and then transformed into a sequence $w(1)...w(L)$ by replacing the 0 by -1, where 'L' is the length of the bit stream and $w(x) \varepsilon \{-1,1\}$ (x=1,...,L). The text watermark embedding and extraction algorithm are discuss in [26]. It is assumed that the original image is available for extraction process

start:
STEP 1: Initialization and inputs

STEP 2: Read the Images
Host Image $\leftarrow$ Kidney.jpg (Medical host image of size 512*512)

STEP 3: Determine DWT coefficients of the host image
//Apply first level DWT on host image
$[LL_1 , LH_1 , HL_1 , HH_1] \leftarrow$ DWT (Host, Haar wavelet);
//Apply second level DWT on host image
$[LL_2 , LH_2 , HL_2 , HH_2] \leftarrow$ DWT (LL_1, Haar wavelet);
//Apply third level DWT on host image
$[LL_3 , LH_3 , HL_3 , HH_3] \leftarrow$ DWT (LL_2, Haar wavelet);

STEP 4: Convert text/personal data to binary bits
Wbinary_bits $\leftarrow$ *binary*(text data of 100 characters);

STEP 5: Apply Hamming/BCH error correcting codes to the *Wbinary_bits*

$Encoded_{binary} bits \leftarrow Hamming \,/\, BCH((Wbinary\_bits)$

STEP 6: Replace '0' bit by '-1' bit in the watermarking bits
$-1bit \leftarrow 0bit;$

STEP 7: Embedding the encoded binary watermark bits in to LL_3 sub-band of the host image

$f'(m, n) = f(m, n)(1 + k \times \text{Encoded}_{\text{binary}}\text{bits}(x))$; $f(m, n)$ and $f'(m, n)$ is the DWT coefficients before and after embedding process respectively

for gain (k) = 0.01 to 0.12 **endif;**

STEP 8: Find the Watermarked Image (containing image and text watermark) using inverse_SVD, inverse_DCT and inverse_DWT respectively

Watermarked_Img ← $(f'(m, n)$, LH_3 , HL_3 , HH_3,Haar wavelet);***end:***

Step 9: For the extraction of text watermark bits, determine DWT coefficients (sub-bands) of possibly distorted decrypted watermarked image

//Apply up to third level DWT on watermarked image

[w_LL1,w_LH1,w_HL1,w_HH1]←DWT(Decrypted_Watermarked, Haar wavelet);

[w_LL2,w_LH2,w_HL2,w_HH2]← DWT(w_LL1,Haar wavelet);

[w_LL3,w_LH3,w_HL3,w_HH3]←DWT(w_LL2, Haar wavelet);

STEP 10: Text/personal information watermark bits extraction

$$W_r(x) = \frac{\left(f_r'(m,n) - f(m,n)\right)}{kf(m,n)}$$; $f_r'(m, n)$ are the DWT coefficients of the received image.

//extracted watermark is taken as positive or negative

$W_e\text{bits}$ ← sign($W_r(x)$);

STEP 4: Apply Hamming or BCH decoder method on $W_e bits$

// modify the watermarking bits by replacing

0 *bit* ← − 1 *bit*; to get the final watermark.

Watermarkbits ← Hamming or BCH decoder $(W_e bits)$

STEP 5: Convert the watermark bits into text to get the original watermark

EPR data ← convertin to Char $(watermarkbits)$

end:

9.4.3 Algorithm 3: Watermarked Image Encryption and Decryption Process

In this section, we discuss the step by step procedure of selective color image encryption as well as decryption process.

STEP 1: The process consist of generation of M×N random number where M*N is the size of image.

for

0.1:200 times

Secret Key (0) ← 3.925 × Secret Key (0) × (1 − Secret Key (0)) ;
Where Secret Key (0) is the value of secret key between 0 to 1.

STEP 2: Use next M×N iterations and find a(m,n), b(m,n) and c(m,n) variables to store the value of Secret Key (0), Secret Key (1)and Secret Key (2) respectively.
a(M, N) ← Secret Key(0);
//Determine b(M,N)
for
0.2:M×N;

$$Secret\ Key(1) \leftarrow 3.925 \times Secret\ Key(1)(1 - Secret\ Key(1))$$

Where initial value of Secret Key (1) = 0.2
b(M, N) ← Secret Key(1);
//Determine c(M,N)
for
0.3:M×N;
Secret Key (2) ← 3.925 × Secret Key (2)(1 − Secret Key (2));
Where initial value of Secret Key (1) = 0.3
$c(M, N) \leftarrow Secret\ Key(\ 2);$

STEP 3: Determine the weight functions
W ← (1 − t)^{2}W$_0$+2t(1-t) W$_1$ + t^{2}W$_2$
Here t= 0.4, W$_0$ = 0.2 , W$_1$ = 0.5 and W$_2$ = 0.3

STEP 4: Determine M×N random number P(m,n)

$$P(m,n) \leftarrow (1-t)^2\ a(m,n) \times W_0 + 2t\ b(m,n) \times W_1 + t^2 c(m,n) \times W_2$$

//For converting into integer value

$$e(M,N) \leftarrow round\ \left(P(M,N) \times 255\right)$$

end;

STEP 5: Selective Encrypt and decrypt process for watermarked image

$$Encryptedwatermarkedimage(M \times N) \leftarrow mod\begin{pmatrix} 0.001 \times Watermarkedimage \\ (M \times N)+(1-0.001) \\ \times e(M,N),256 \end{pmatrix}$$

//for decryption process generate the e(m,n) random number from secret key as done in previous steps.

$$DecryptedWatermarkedimage(M \times N) \leftarrow \frac{(EncryptedWatermarkedimage(M \times N) - (1-0.001) \times e(M,N)}{0.001}$$

end:

9.5 Experimental Results and Performance Analysis

The performance of proposed hybrid watermarking method is based on DWT, DCT, SVD, BPNN and Selective encryption on watermarked image has been investigated. Different color/gray images from Internet were tested as cover and watermark image of different size was used to demonstrate the experimental results. The visual quality of the hidden watermark and the robustness of the extracted image watermark were evaluated by determining PSNR and NC values respectively. The robustness of the text/personal information watermarks is evaluated by determining BER value. In the proposed technique, cover image, image watermark and text watermark of size 512×512, 128×128 and 100 characters respectively are used for experimental purpose. It is quite apparent that size of the watermark affects quality of the watermarked image. However, degradation in quality of the watermarked image will not be observable if the size of watermark (total size in case of multiple watermarking) is small. The security of the host image and watermarks is enhanced by applying the selective encryption on the watermarked image which reduces the computational requirements in e-health applications. The robustness (determining NC and BER) of the proposed method against different known attacks was compared with the robustness offered by reported methods [18–22]. In addition, imperceptibility (determining PSNR), capacity and Encryption/decryption time are also compared with other reported techniques. Figures 9.3 and 9.4 show the different cover and watermark images, respectively.

Figure 9.5 show the personal information considered as text watermarks. Figure 9.6 show the corresponding watermarked images. Figures 9.7 and 9.8 show the corresponding selective encrypted and decrypted watermarked images respectively. Figures 9.9 and 9.10 show the extracted different watermarks without and with using BPNN respectively. Figure 9.11a–c show the Histogram of the watermarked, selectively encrypted watermarked and decrypted watermarked image, respectively.

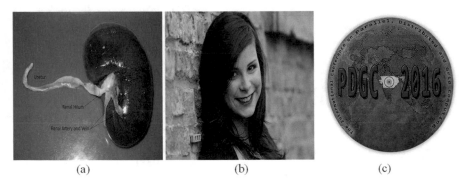

(a)   (b)   (c)

Fig. 9.3 Cover Images (**a**) kidney (**b**) Lena and (**c**) PDGC_logo

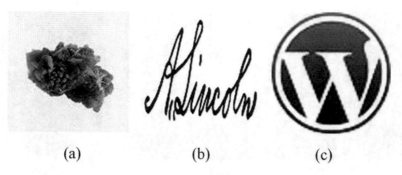

(a)   (b)   (c)

Fig. 9.4 Watermark images (**a**) stone (**b**) signature (**c**) logo

Fig. 9.5 Personal
information using as text
watermark

Personal Information:
Name: Dr.AmitKumarSingh
Father's Name: ShriShivrajSingh
Person Identity Number: BXRTG5264D
Age: 36Y
Gender: Male
Contact Address: Deptt.of_CSE_JUITWaknaghat, Solan
Blood group: B+
Medical Reports: OPD_15_HighFever

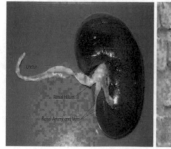
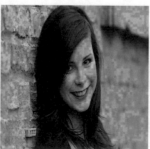
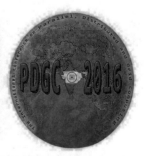

Fig. 9.6 Corresponding watermarked images

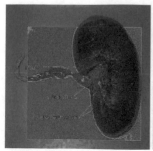
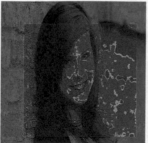
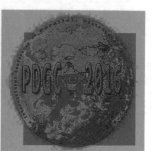

Fig. 9.7 Corresponding selective encrypted watermarked images

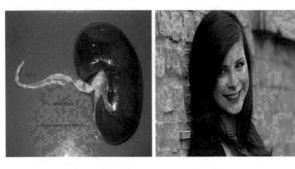
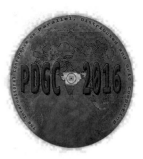

Fig. 9.8 Corresponding selective decrypted watermarked images

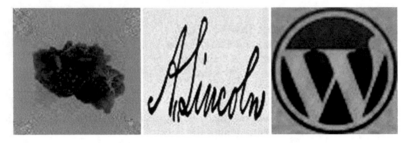

Fig. 9.9 Extracted watermark images without using BPNN

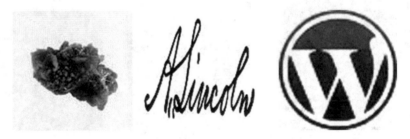

Fig. 9.10 Extracted watermark images using BPNN

Personal Information:
Name: Dr.AmitKumarSingh
Father's Name: ShriShivrajSingh
Person Identity Number: BXRTG5264D
Age: 36Y
Gender: Male
Contact Address: Deptt.of_CSE_JUITWaknaghat, Solan
Blood group: B+
Medical Reports: OPD_15_HighFever

The performance of the proposed techniques is determined in Tables 9.4, 9.5, 9.6, 9.7, 9.8, 9.9, 9.10, 9.11, 9.12, and 9.13. Table 9.4 shows the PSNR, NC (with

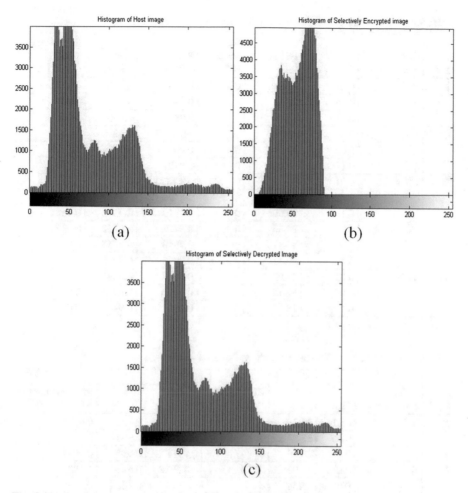

Fig. 9.11 Histogram for (**a**) watermarked image (**b**) encrypted and (**c**) decrypted watermarked image

and without using the BPNN) and BER performance of the proposed technique at different gain for YCbCr color model. In this table, the watermarks (image and text) are embedding in to the different components of the color model is investigated. With reference to this table, the 'Y' component of the YCbCr model is suitable for the embedded both watermarks.

The highest NC value is 0.9965 at gain factor = 0.1 using BPNN. However, the NC value is 0.9948 without using the BPNN at the same gain factor. The minimum NC value is 0.8737 at gain factor = 0.01 using BPNN. However, the NC value is 0.8464 without using the BPNN at the same gain factor. The maximum PSNR value is 34.84 dB for the Y component at gain = 0.01. However, the minimum PSNR value

Table 9.4 Performance of YCbCr model (kidney, stone, 40 characters)

SN	Color component	Gain	PSNR (dB)	BER using BCH	NC Without BPNN	With BPNN	Improvements in NC values (%)
1.	YY	0.01	34.84	0	0.8464	0.8737	0.0312
		0.05	32.21	0	0.9945	0.9959	0.0014
		0.1	28.68	0	0.9948	0.9965	0.0017
2.	CbCb	0.01	34.86	0	−0.4827	0.5214	1.9257
		0.05	32.66	0	0.9037	0.9736	0.0717
		0.1	29.71	0	0.9137	0.9616	0.0498
3.	CrCr	0.01	34.90	0	−0.2392	0.4585	1.5217
		0.05	33.11	0	0.8796	0.9152	0.0388
		0.1	29.99	0	0.8719	0.9318	0.0642
4.	YCr	0.01	34.86	0	0.8428	0.8712	0.0325
		0.05	32.51	0	0.9940	0.9955	0.0015
		0.1	29.11	0	0.9948	0.9965	0.0017
5.	YCb	0.01	34.83	0	0.8277	0.8575	0.0347
		0.05	32.16	0	0.9940	0.9955	0.0015
		0.1	28.91	0	0.9947	0.9965	0.0018

Table 9.5 Performance of YIQ model (kidney, stone, 40 characters)

SN	Color component	Gain	PSNR (dB)	BER using BCH	NC Without BPNN	With BPNN	Improvements in NC values (%)
1.	YY	0.01	34.88	0	0.76	0.8013	0.0515
		0.05	32.88	0	0.9929	0.9947	0.0018
		0.1	29.89	0	0.9911	0.9958	0.0047
2.	II	0.01	34.97	23.21	−0.5928	0.5930	1.999
		0.05	34.54	0	0.6109	0.7220	0.1538
		0.1	33.35	0	0.8524	0.8909	0.0432
3.	QQ	0.01	34.98	41.43	−0.2257	0.4580	1.4927
		0.05	34.34	18.57	0.9111	0.9467	0.0376
		0.1	32.54	1.0714	0.9425	0.9748	0.0331
4.	YI	0.01	34.94	24.64	0.7718	0.8107	0.0479
		0.05	34.05	0	0.9931	0.9948	0.0017
		0.1	32.40	0	0.9907	0.9956	0.0049
5.	YQ	0.01	34.96	44.28	0.7593	0.7988	0.0494
		0.05	34.15	22.14	0.9916	0.9935	0.0019
		0.1	32.65	0	0.9907	0.9955	0.0048

Table 9.6 Performance of YCbCr model for different size of text watermark

SN	Text watermark size	Gain factor	PSNR (dB)	BER		NC		Improvements in NC values (%)
				Hamming	BCH	Without BPNN	With BPNN	
1.	20	0.01	34.88	0.7143	0	0.8364	0.8649	0.0329
		0.05	33.64	0.7143	0	0.9944	0.9956	0.0012
		0.1	29.68	0	0	0.9945	0.9963	0.0018
2.	40	0.01	34.84	0.3571	0	0.8464	0.8737	0.0312
		0.05	32.21	0	0	0.9945	0.9959	0.0014
		0.1	28.68	0	0	0.9948	0.9965	0.0017
3.	64	0.01	34.78	0.2232	0	0.8572	0.8833	0.0295
		0.05	31.65	0	0	0.9941	0.9959	0.0018
		0.1	27.77	0	0	0.9949	0.9961	0.0012
4.	100	0.01	34.74	0.1429	0.1021	0.5827	0.7445	0.2173
		0.05	31.03	0	0	0.9939	0.9955	0.0016
		0.1	26.79	0	0	0.9937	0.9961	0.0024

Table 9.7 Performance of YCbCr model at different gain factors

SN	Gain factor	PSNR (dB)	BER		NC		Improvements in NC values (%)
			Using Hamming code	Using BCH code	Without BPNN	With BPNN	
1.	0.01	34.78	0.2232	0	0.8572	0.8833	0.0295
2.	0.02	34.25	0	0	0.9771	0.9836	0.0066
3.	0.05	31.65	0	0	0.9941	0.9959	0.0018
4.	0.07	29.94	0	0	0.9950	0.9962	0.0012
5.	0.08	29.17	0	0	0.9949	0.9960	0.0011
6.	0.1	27.77	0	0	0.9949	0.9961	0.0012
7.	0.12	26.57	0	0	0.9947	0.9962	0.0015

Table 9.8 Performance of YCbCr model for different cover and watermark images at gain 0.07 (64 characters)

SN	Cover image	Watermark image	PSNR (dB)	BER(%) using BCH	NC		Improvements in NC values (%)
					Without BPNN	With BPNN	
1.	Brain	Stone	28.54	7.366	0.9659	0.9808	0.0151
2.	Intestine	Stone	28.96	1.5625	0.9862	0.9934	0.0072
3.	Heart	Stone	28.80	0	0.9840	0.9950	0.0110
4.	Patient	Stone	28.81	0	0.9839	0.9946	0.0107
5.	JUIT_logo	Logo	28.92	39.06	0.8272	0.8452	0.0236
6.	PDGC_logo	Logo	27.70	0	0.9940	0.9964	0.0024
7.	Magzine_cover	Logo	27.67	0	0.9980	0.9985	0.0005
8.	Lena	Signature	29.36	0	0.9968	0.9987	0.0019
9.	Ian	Signature	30.96	0	0.9941	0.9979	0.0038
10.	Doctor	Signature	28.07	0	0.9786	0.9946	0.0160

Table 9.9 Performance of YCbCr model for different attacks at gain 0.07 (64 characters)

SN	Attacks	BER	NC Without BPNN	With BPNN	Improvements in NC values (%)
1.	JPEG (QF = 5)	0	0.7087	0.7782	0.0893
2.	JPEG (QF = 10)	0	0.9627	0.9819	0.0195
3.	JPEG (QF = 30)	0	0.9915	0.9945	0.0030
4.	JPEG (QF = 70)	0	0.9906	0.9936	0.0030
5.	JPEG (QF = 90)	0	0.9945	0.9957	0.0012
6.	Salt & Peppers (d = 0.02)	0	0.6808	0.7564	0.0999
7.	Salt & Peppers (d = 0.01)	0	0.8161	0.8670	0.0587
8.	Salt & Peppers (d = 0.005)	0	0.9095	0.9434	0.0359
9.	Salt & Peppers (d = 0.08)	0.4464	0.4510	0.5918	0.2379
10.	Gaussian (M = 0, v = 0.01)	0	0.6151	0.7033	0.1254
11.	Gaussian (M = 0, v = 0.005)	0	0.7317	0.7952	0.0798
12.	Gaussian (M = 0.01, v = 0.08)	2.9018	0.3614	0.5266	0.3137
13.	Speckle (v = 0.05)	0	0.5775	0.6854	0.1574
14.	Speckle (v = 0.1)	1.5625	0.4737	0.6205	0.2365
15.	Speckle (v = 0.02)	0	0.7331	0.8021	0.0860
16.	Average Filter [2 2]	0	0.8071	0.8478	0.0480
17.	Average Filter [3 3]	0	−0.0106	0.5739	1.0184
18.	Gaussian Low pass Filter [3 3]	0	0.9304	0.9362	0.00619
19.	Gaussian Low pass Filter [2 2]	0	0.8071	0.8474	0.0475
20.	Gaussian Low pass Filter [4 4]	0	0.7547	0.8172	0.0764
21.	Motion Blur (len = 10, Theta = 2)	0	0.3146	0.5799	0.4574
22.	Crop (5%)	53.79	0.1605	0.3331	0.5281
23.	Resize (scale = 0.85)	0	0.7803	0.8331	0.0633
24.	Rotate (5°)	45.76	0.3512	0.7154	0.5090
25.	JPEG (QF = 90) + Salt & Peppers (d = 0.005)	0	0.9043	0.9404	0.0383
26.	JPEG (QF = 90) + Gaussian (M = 0, v = 0.005)	0	0.7184	0.7865	0.0865
27.	JPEG (QF = 70) + Speckle (v = 0.02)	0	0.7333	0.8017	0.0853
28.	Salt & Peppers(d = 0.002) + Gaussian (M = 0,v = 0.005)	0	0.6978	0.7673	0.09057
29.	Salt & Peppers (d = 0.005) + Speckle (v = 0.02)	0	0.6975	0.7714	0.0957
30.	Gaussian (M = 0, v = 0.005) + Speckle (v = 0.02)	0	0.6049	0.6987	0.1342

is 28.68 dB for the same color component at the gain = 0.1. Here the BER value has been obtained as '0' for the Y component at the selected gain factors (0.01 to 0.1).

Table 9.5 shows the PSNR, NC (with and without using the BPNN) and BER performance of the proposed technique at different gain for YIQ color model. In this table, the watermarks (image and text) are embedding in to the different components

Table 9.10 Encryption and Decryption time for different cover

SN	Encrypted part (%)	Kidney (512 * 512)-stone (128 * 128)		PDGC_logo (512 * 512)-W logo (128 * 128)		Lena (512 * 512)-Signature (128 * 128)	
		ENC time (second)	DEC time (second)	ENC time (second)	DEC time (second)	ENC time (second)	DEC time (second)
1.	10%	0.3900	0.6396	0.4056	0.6396	0.3900	0.6396
2.	20%	0.4212	0.8268	0.4368	0.5928	0.4212	0.6552
3.	50%	0.5928	0.7488	0.5772	0.6084	0.5928	0.8112
4.	75%	0.8424	0.6396	0.8580	0.6552	0.8424	0.6240
5.	78%	0.9672	0.6240	0.8736	0.6708	0.8892	0.6864
6.	100%	1.2168	0.6864	1.2324	0.6552	1.2480	0.6708

Table 9.11 The performance comparison under NC with watermark size of 128 × 128

Attacks	NC values		
	Ghafoor et al. [18]	Proposed method	Improvements in NC values (%)
Histogram equilization	0.8381	0.9028	0.0716
Rotation (2°)	0.8534	0.9081	0.0602
Gaussian noise(M = 0, V = 0.001)	0.8287	0.9663	0.1423
Scaling	0.8393	0.8434	0.0048
Cropping (2%)	0.4918	0.9317	0.4721
Median Filtering [2 2]	0.8307	0.8707	0.0459
Salt & Peppers (d = 0.01)	0.8227	0.867	0.0510
JPEG (QF = 20)	–	0.9919	–

of the color model is investigated. Refereeing this table, the 'Y' component of the YIQ model is suitable for the embedding both watermarks. The highest NC value is 0.9958 at gain factor = 0.1 using BPNN. However, the NC value is 0.9948 without using the BPNN at the same gain factor. The minimum NC value is 0.8013 at gain factor = 0.01 using BPNN. However, the NC value is 0.76 without using the BPNN at the same gain factor. The maximum PSNR value is 34.88 dB for the Y component of the YIQ model at gain = 0.01. However, the minimum PSNR value is 29.89 dB for the same color component at the gain = 0.1. Here the BER value has been obtained as '0' for the Y component at the selected gain factors (0.01–0.1). Based on the results as obtained in Tables 9.4 and 9.5, it is noticed that the YCbCr model is perform better than YIQ model, where the Y component of the model is suitable for embedding the watermarks.

Table 9.6 shows that PSNR, BER (with Hamming and BCH error correcting codes) and NC (with and without using the BPNN) performance of the proposed hybrid technique at different gain factors for different size (20–100 characters) of text watermark. For the maximum size of watermark (100 characters), the highest NC value is 0.9961 at gain factor = 0.1 using BPNN. However, the NC value is

Table 9.12 The performance comparison under NC watermark size of 64 × 64

SN	Attacks	Xing et al. [17]	Santhi et al. [19]	Zhao et al. [20]	Xiong et al. [21]	Shi et al. [22]	Proposed method
1	JPEG (QF = 80)	0.9648	–	0.9767	0.9844	–	0.9882
2	JPEG (QF = 70)	0.9537	–	–	0.9163	–	0.9878
3	JPEG (QF = 60)	0.9361	–	–	0.8564	–	0.9854
4	JPEG (QF = 50)	0.91	–	–	–	–	0.9835
5	JPEG (QF = 40)	0.8776	–	0.9252	–	–	0.9819
6	JPEG (QF = 30)	–	–	–	–	0.9132	0.9865
7	JPEG (QF = 20)	–	0.766	0.8635	–	0.7586	0.9872
8	Salt & Peppers (d = 0.01)	–	–	0.5473	–	0.7331	0.9579
9	Salt & Peppers (d = 0.02)	–	–	0.4657	–	–	0.8696
10	Salt & Peppers (d = 0.005)	–	–	–	0.9709	0.8016	0.9744
11	Gaussian noise (M = 0, V = 0.01)	–	–	0.5473	–	–	0.8184
12	Gaussian noise(M = 0, V = 0.02)	–	–	0.4657	–	–	0.674
13	Resize 1.3x	0.9714	0.986	–	–	–	0.9906
14	Resize 1.1x	0.9221	–	–	–	–	0.9824
15	Resize 0.8x	0.9443	–	–	–	–	0.9738
16	Resize 0.7x	0.9058	–	–	–	–	0.9624
17	Rotation with cropping (0.25°)	0.895	–	–	–	–	0.9741
18	Rotation with cropping (0.5°)	0.8898	–	–	–	–	0.9297
19	Rotation with cropping (1°)	0.8536	–	–	–	–	0.9238
20	Rotation with cropping (2°)	0.9322	–	–	–	–	0.9254
21	Rotation (5°)	–	0.577	–	–	–	0.8269
22	Median filtering [2 2]	0.8773	–	–	–	–	0.979
23	Color contrast	–	0.93	–	–	–	0.9246
24	Crop	–	0.822	–	–	–	0.9859
25	Speckle	–	–	–	0.9747	–	0.9883
26	Gaussian lowpass filter ([5 5], 0.5)	–	–	–	–	0.9824	0.9865

0.9937 without using the BPNN at the same gain factor. The minimum NC value is 0.7445 at gain factor = 0.01 using BPNN. However, the NC value is 0.5827 without using the BPNN at the same gain factor. Referring this table, the maximum BER value is 0.1429 at gain factor = 0.01 using Hamming code.

Table 9.13 Visual quality of the watermarked by subjective methods	Gain factors	PSNR (dB)	Quality of watermarked image
	0.01	34.78	Very good imperceptible
	0.07	29.94	Good imperceptible
	0.12	26.57	Bad imperceptible

However, the BER value is 0.1021 at the same gain using BCH error correcting code. The BER value (using BCH code) is found to be 0 for other size of watermarks. Table 9.7 shows that PSNR, BER (with Hamming and BCH error correcting codes) and NC (with and without using the BPNN) performance of the proposed technique at different gain factors for the text watermark size of 64 characters. The highest NC value is 0.9962 at gain factor = 0.12 using BPNN. However, the NC value is 0.9947 without using the BPNN at the same gain factor. The minimum NC value is 0.8833 at gain factor = 0.01 using BPNN. However, the NC value is 0.8572 without using the BPNN at the same gain factor. Referring this table, the maximum BER value is 0.2232 at gain factor = 0.01 using Hamming code. However, the BER value is '0' at the same gain using BCH error correcting code. The BER value (using BCH code) is found to be '0' at different gain.

Table 9.8 shows that PSNR, BER (with BCH error correcting codes) and NC (with and without using the BPNN) performance of the proposed technique at gain factors = 0.07 for the different host and image watermark. Here, the size of the text watermark is 64 characters. Referring Table 9.8 it can be inferred that the NC values vary in the range from 0.8452 to 0.9987 using BPNN. However, NC values vary in the range from 0.8272 to 0.9980 without using BPNN. The maximum and BER value is 39.06% for '*JUIT*' logo considered as host image. However, the minimum BER value is 0 for others host images except for the Brain and Intestine images. Referring this table, it is observed that the PSNR values vary in the range from 27.67 to 30.96 dB using image and text watermark size of 128 × 128 and 64 characters respectively. The highest NC value is 0.9962 at gain factor = 0.12 using BPNN. However, the NC value is 0.9947 without using the BPNN at the same gain factor. The minimum NC value is 0.8833 at gain factor = 0.01 using BPNN. However, the NC value is 0.8572 without using the BPNN at the same gain factor. In this table, the maximum BER value is 0.2232 at gain factor = 0.01 using Hamming code. However, the BER value is 0 at the same gain using BCH error correcting code. The BER value (using BCH code) is found to be '0' at different gain. The NC and BER performance of the proposed hybrid watermarking method has been extensively evaluated against different known attacks in Table 9.9. Referring this table it can be inferred that the NC values vary in the range from 0.3331 (for cropping attacks) to 0.9957 (for JPEG QF = 90%) using BPNN. However, NC values vary in the range from −0.0106 (Average Filter [3 3]) to 0.9945 (JPEG QF = 90) without using BPNN. In this table, the BER = 0 is obtained for all considered attacks except Salt & Peppers (d = 0.08), Gaussian (M = 0.01, v = 0.08), Speckle (v = 0.1), Crop (5%) and Rotate (5°) attacks. Referring this table it can be observed that the NC and BER performance of the proposed technique highly depends on noise variations.

Table 9.10 shows that the encryption and decryption time for different cover and watermark image using selective encryption technique. Referring this table it can be observed that the encryption/decryption time highly depends on encrypted part of the watermarked/cover image. In the proposed technique, 78% important part of the watermarked image is encrypted. The maximum and minimum encrypted time is 0.9672 and 0.8736 for Kidney/stone and PDGC_logo/logo respectively. However, maximum and minimum decrypted time is 0.6864 and 0.6240 for Lena/Signature and Kidney/stone respectively.

The NC performance of the proposed method is compared with other reported techniques (using watermark size of 128×128) in Table 9.11. Referring this table it can be inferred that the NC values as obtained by Ghafoor and Imran [18] vary in the range from 0.4918 to 0.8534 at gain factor 'α' = 0.07. However, the NC values as obtained by proposed technique vary in the range from 0.8434 to 0.9919 at same gain. In addition, the table show that the proposed method offer up to 0.4721% in NC performance than reported technique [18]. Table 9.12 shows the NC performance of the proposed method is compared with other reported techniques (using watermark size of 64 × 64) [19–22]. Referring the table it can be inferred that the NC values as obtained by proposed method vary in the range from 0.6740 to 0.9906 at gain factor 'α' = 0.07. The maximum NC value has been obtained by the proposed method is 0.9906 with image Resize attacks (1.3 × 1.3). However, the minimum NC value is 0.6740 for Gaussian noise (M = 0, V = 0.02). In this table, the maximum NC value has been obtained by the Xing and Tan [17], Santhi and Thangavelu [19], Zhao and Dang [20], Xiong [21] and Shi et al. [22] is 0.9767, 0.9714, 0.9862, 0.9844 and 0.9824, respectively.

Further, the NC performance of the proposed method is compared with the methods reported in [17, 18, 19, 20, 21, 22] is presented in Figs. 9.12, 9.13, 9.14, 9.15, 9.16, 9.17, respectively. In recent era, medical image processing is also a great important for efficient diagnosis purpose [47]. Moreover, we have examined the visual quality of the watermarked image by subjective method [48] in Table 9.13. This method involve an expert from medical fields and some students were examined the visual quality if the watermarked image. In this table, it is observed that the image is suitable for the medical diagnosis purpose at the considered gain factor except for gain = 0.12.

From the above extensive discussion, the proposed method offers the optimum trade-off between major benchmark parameters (robustness, visual quality, capacity and security). In addition, the method offer better performance than other reported techniques [18–22]. The performance of the proposed method highly depends of gain, noise level and size of the watermarks.

9.6   Summary and Future Directions

In this chapter, we have presented a robust and secure multiple watermarking method using combination of DWT, DCT, SVD, selective encryption, error correcting codes, and Neural Network. The method has been found potentially useful in

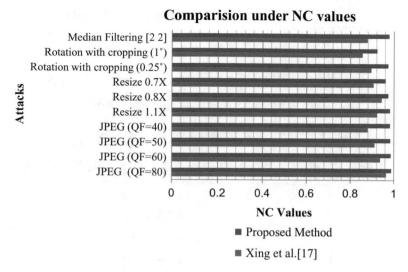

Fig. 9.12 NC performance comparison with Xing and Tan [17]

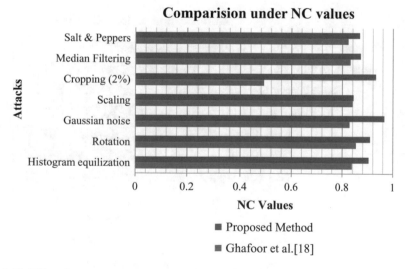

Fig. 9.13 NC performance comparison with Ghafoor and Imran [18]

achieving enhanced robustness as well as security of the watermark which can be gainfully extracted in medical as well as other applications of secure document dissemination. In addition, the proposed method offer optimal trade-off between robustness, perceptual quality of the cover image, amount of embedded data and security of the watermark embedded into digital images. Tables 9.4 and 9.5 show the PSNR, NC (with and without using the BPNN) and BER performance of the proposed technique at different gain for YCbCr and YIQ color model, respectively.

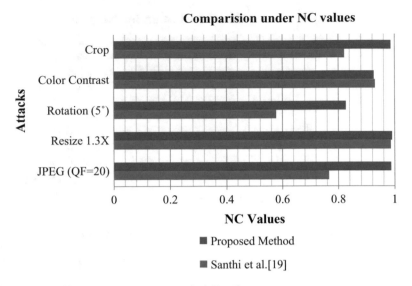

Fig. 9.14 NC performance comparison with Santhi and Thangavelu [19]

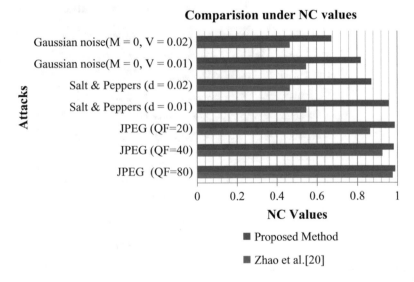

Fig. 9.15 NC performance comparison with Zhao and Dang [20]

With refernce to Tables 9.5 and 9.6, it is established that the NC performance of the proposed techniques is enhanced up to 1.9257% and 1.999% for YCbCr and YIQ color model respectively using BPNN method. Table 9.6 shows that PSNR, BER and NC performance of the proposed hybrid technique at different gain factors for different size (20–100 characters) of text watermark. As inferred from this Table, the proposed method offered up to 0.2173% enhancements in robustness (determine by NC value) using BPNN method.

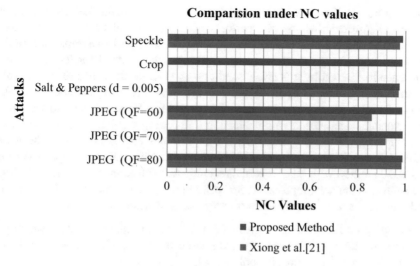

Fig. 9.16 NC performance comparison with Xiong [21]

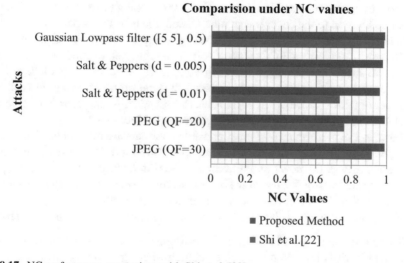

Fig. 9.17 NC performance comparison with Shi et al. [22]

The PSNR, BER and NC performance of the proposed technique at different gain factors for the text/personal information watermark size of 64 characters is evaluated in Table 9.7. Referring this Table it can be inferred that the NC performance is enhanced up to 0.0295% using BPNN. In addition, the BER performance of the proposed method is investigated with two different error correcting codes. It is found the BCH error correcting code performs better than Hamming code. Table 9.8 shows that PSNR, BER and NC performance of the proposed technique at gain factors = 0.07 for the different host and image watermark. Referring this Table it can be inferred that the NC performance is enhanced up to 0.0236% using BPNN. The NC and BER performance of the proposed hybrid watermarking method has been extensively evaluated against different known attacks in Table 9.9. With reference to this Table, it is established that the NC performance of the proposed techniques is enhanced up to 1.0184% using BPNN training method. Table 9.10 shows that the encryption and decryption time for different cover and watermark image using selective encryption technique. Referring this table it can be observed that the encryption/decryption time highly depends encrypted part of the water-marked image. Tables 9.11 and 9.12 show the NC performance comparison of the proposed method with other reported techniques. With reference to these Tables, it is established that the proposed method offer better performance than other reported techniques. The main contribution of the work is identified as follows:

1. The proposed cost effective method embedding multiple watermark which provides the extra level of security and reduce storage/bandwidth requirements in many discussed multimedia applications.
2. The work further addresses the issue of channel noise distortions leading to faulty watermark in different applications. The proposed method solved this issue by using BCH and Hamming ECCs for encoding the text watermark before embedding in to the cover image. In addition, the robustness performance of the image and text watermark is enhanced by using the Back Propagation Neural Network (BPNN) and ECCs respectively. The suggested method is robust against known attacks without significant degradation of the cover image quality. Based on experimental results, it is established that the proposed technique achieved superior performance in respect of robustness, capacity, and security with acceptable visual quality as compared to other reported techniques.
3. Further, the performance of the proposed watermarking method has been investigated by applying selective encryption on watermarked data which enhanced the security of the cover and watermarks data. In addition, selective encryption is computationally fast for large size of multimedia contents to offers confidentiality of digital contents for various multimedia applications.
4. The proposed method also addresses personal/health data management issues.

Therefore, the proposed method is providing potential solutions in prevention of personal identity theft and unauthorized content sharing on online social networks/open channel for various applications. Further work can be carried out to minimize the computational complexity of the proposed techniques for color image water-marking. The computational complexity of the proposed watermarking method can be minimizing by selecting and exploring the other wavelet instead of DWT.

In future, the performance analysis of the method can also be examined with directional transform techniques, biometrics, turbo code and extended for their application to video watermarking.

References

1. T. H-The, O. Banos, S. Lee, Y. Yoon, T. Le-Tien, A novel watermarking scheme for image authentication in social networks, in Proceedings of the 9th International Conference on Ubiquitous Information Management and Communication, BALI, Indonesia, Article No. 48, 2015. DOI:10.1145/2701126.2701237
2. A.K. Singh, B. Kumar, M. Dave, S.P. Ghrera, A. Mohan et al., Digital image watermarking: techniques and emerging applications, in *Handbook of Research on Modern Cryptographic Solutions for Computer and Cyber Security*, ed. by B.B. Gupta (IGI Global, Hershey, 2016), pp. 246–272
3. Z. Zhang, B.B. Gupta, Social media security and trustworthiness: overview and new direction, in *Future Generation Computer Systems*, (Elsevier, 2016)
4. A. Zigomitros, A. Papageorgiou, C. Patsakis, Social network content management through watermarking, in 11th International Conference on Trust, Security and Privacy in Computing and Communications, Liverpool, pp. 1381–1386, 2012
5. S. Iftikhar, M. Kamran, E.U. Munir, S.U. Khan, A reversible watermarking technique for social network data sets for enabling data trust in cyber, physical, and social computing. IEEE Syst. J. **11**(1), 197–206 (2017)
6. M. Terry, Medical identity theft and telemedicine security. Telemed. e-Health **15**(10), 928–932 (2009)
7. D. Bowman., http://www.fiercehealthit.com/story/researchers-use-digital-watermarks-protect-medical-images, 2012
8. M. Ollove., www.usatoday.com/story/.../stateline-identity-thefts-medical.../5279351, *2014*
9. A.K. Singh, M. Dave, A. Mohan, Robust and secure multiple watermarking in wavelet domain. A special issue on advanced signal processing technologies and systems for healthcare applications. J. Med. Imaging Health Inf. **5**(2), 406–414 (2015)
10. A.K. Singh, M. Dave, A. Mohan, Wavelet based image watermarking: futuristic concepts in information security. Proc. Nat. Acad. Sci. India Sect. A: Phys. Sci. **84**(3), 345–359 (2014)
11. S.P. Mohanty, Watermarking of digital images, M.S. Thesis, Indian Institute of Science, India, 1999
12. M.C. Wolak, Digital watermarking, in *Preliminary Proposal*, (Nova Southeastern University, United States, 2000)
13. N. Nikolaidis, I. Pitas, Digital image watermarking: an overview. IEEE Int. Conf. Multimedia Comput. Syst. **1**, 1–6 (1999)
14. I.J. Cox, M.L. Miller, The first 50 years of electronic watermarking. EURASIP J. Adv. Signal Proc. **2002**, 126–132 (2002)
15. A Kannammal, S Subha Rani, Two level security for medical images using watermarking/encryption algorithms. Int. J. Imaging Syst. Technol. **24**(1), 111–120 (2014)
16. A. Al-Haj, A. Amer, Secured telemedicine using region-based watermarking with tamper localization. J. Digit. Imaging **27**(6), 737–750 (2014)
17. Y. Xing, J. Tan, A color image watermarking scheme resistant against geometrical attacks. Radioengineering **19**(1), 62–67 (2010)
18. A. Ghafoor, M. Imran, A non-blind color image watermarking scheme resistent against geometric attacks. Radioengineering **21**(4), 1246–1251 (2012)
19. V. Santhi, A. Thangavelu, DC coefficients based watermarking technique for color images using singular value decomposition. Int. J. Comput. Electr. Eng. **3**(1), 8–16 (2011)
20. M. Zhao, Y. Dang, Color image copyright protection digital watermarking algorithm based on DWT & DCT, in 4th International Conference on Wireless Communications, Networking and Mobile Computing, Dalian, pp. 1–4, 12–14 Oct 2008
21. X. Xiong, A new robust color image watermarking scheme based on 3D-DCT. World J. Eng. Technol. **3**, 177–183 (2015)
22. H. Shi, F. Lv, Y. Cao, A blind watermarking technique for color image based on SVD with circulation. J. Software **9**(7), 1749–1756 (2014)

23. N. Ramamurthy, S. Varadarajan, The robust digital image watermarking scheme with back propagation neural network in DWT domain. Int. J. Comput. Sci. Network Security **13**(1), 111–117 (2013)
24. N.V. Dharwadkar, B.B. Amberker, An Efficient non blind watermarking scheme for colour images using discrete wavelet transformation. Int. J. Comput. Appl. **2**(3), 60–66 (2010)
25. A. Sharma, A.K. Singh, S.P. Ghrera, Robust and secure multiple watermarking technique for medical images. Wirel. Pers. Commun. **92**(4), 1611–1624 (2017)
26. A. Zear, A.K. Singh, P. Kumar, A proposed secure multiple watermarking technique based on DWT, DCT and SVD for application in medicine. Multimedia Tools Appl. (2016). doi:10.1007/s11042-016-3862-8
27. R. Pandey, A.K. Singh, B. Kumar, A. Mohan, Iris based secure NROI multiple eye image watermarking for teleophthalmology. Multimedia Tools Appl. **75**(22), 14381–14397 (2016)
28. S.J.J. Mary, C.S. Christopher, S.S.A. Joe, Novel scheme for compressed image authentication using LSB watermarking and EMRC6 encryption. Circuits Syst. **7**, 1722–1733 (2016)
29. G. Badshah, S.-C. Liew, J.M. Zain, M. Ali, Watermark compression in medical image watermarking using lempel-ziv-welch (LZW) lossless compression technique. J. Digit. Imaging **29**(2), 216–225 (2016)
30. J M Guo and H Prasetyo, False-positive-free SVD-based image watermarking, J. Vis. Commun. Image Represent., **25**(5), 1149–1163 (2014).
31. F.N. Thakkar, V.K. Srivastava, A blind medical image watermarking: DWT-SVD based robust and secure approach for telemedicine applications. Multimedia Tools Appl. **76**(3), 3669–3697 (2017)
32. K. Wu, W. Yan, J. Du, A robust dual digital-image watermarking technique, in International Conference on Computational Intelligence and Security Workshop, pp. 668–671, 2007
33. C. Chemak, M.S. Bouhlel, J.C. Lapayre, A new scheme of robust image watermarking: the double watermarking algorithm, in Proceedings of the 2007 Summer Computer Simulation Conference, San Diego, California, USA, pp. 1201–1208, 2007
34. H. Shen, B. Chen, From single watermark to dual watermark: a new approach for image watermarking. Comput. Electr. Eng. **38**(5), 1310–1324 (2012)
35. A. Singh, A. Tayal, Choice of wavelet from wavelet families for DWT–DCT–SVD image watermarking. Int. J. Comput. Appl. **48**(17), 9–14 (2012)
36. M.I. Khan, M.M. Rahman, M.I.H. Sarker, Digital watermarking for image authentication based on combined DCT, DWT, and SVD transformation. Int. J. Comput. Sci. **10**(5), 223–230 (2013)
37. A. Srivastava, P. Saxena, DWT-DCT-SVD based semi blind image watermarking using middle frequency band. IOSR J. Comput. Eng. **12**(2), 63–66 (2013)
38. N.J. Harish, B.B.S. Kumar, A. Kusagur, Hybrid robust watermarking techniques based on DWT, DCT, and SVD. Int. J. Adv. Electr. Electr. Eng. **2**(5), 137–143 (2013)
39. I.J. Cox, J. Kilian, F.T. Leighton, T. Shamoon, Secure spread spectrum watermarking for multimedia. IEEE Trans. Image Process. **6**(12), 1673–1687 (1997)
40. B.L. Gunjal, R.R. Manthalkar, An overview of transform domain robust digital image watermarking algorithms. J. Emerg. Trends Comput. Inf. Sci. **2**(1), 13–16 (2011)
41. F. Chen, H. He, Y. Huo, H. Wang, Self-recovery fragile watermarking scheme with variable watermark payload, in Proceedings of the 10th international conference on Digital-Forensics and Watermarking, Atlantic City, NY, pp. 142–155, 2011
42. N.H. Divecha, N.N. Jani, Image watermarking algorithm using DCT, DWT and SVD. Proc. Natl. Conf. Innov. Paradigms Eng. Technol. **10**, 13–16 (2012)
43. K.A. Navas, A.M. Cheriyan, M. Lekshmi, S.A. Tampy, M. Sasikumar, DWT–DCT–SVD based watermarking, in Proceedings of the 3rd International Conference on Communication Systems Software and Middleware and Workshop, Bangalore, pp. 271–274, 2008
44. B. Wang, J. Ding, Q. Wen, X. Liao, C. Liu, An Image watermarking algorithm based on DWT DCT and SVD. IEEE Int. Conf. Network Infrastruct. Dig. Content, Beijing, 1034–1038 (2009)

45. A Giakoumaki, S Pavlopoulos, and D Koutsouris, "Multiple image watermarking applied to health information management", IEEE Trans. Inf. Technol. Biomed., Vol. 10, No. 4, pp. 722-732, 2006.
46. X. Liu, A.M. Eskicioglu, Selective encryption of multimedia content in distribution networks: challenges and new directions, in 2nd International Conference on communication, internet and information technology, pp. 527–533, 2003
47. M. Alsmirat, Y. Jararweh, M. Al-Ayyoub, M.A. Shehab, B.B. Gupta, Accelerating compute intensive medical imaging segmentation algorithms using GPUs. Multimedia Tools Appl. (2016). doi:10.1007/s11042-016-3884-2
48. A.K. Singh, Some new techniques of improved wavelet domain watermarking for medical images, Ph.D. Thesis, Department of Computer Engineering, NIT Kurukshetra, Haryana, India, 2015

Chapter 10
State-of-the-Art Techniques of Image Watermarking: New Trends and Future Challenges

Amit Kumar Singh, Basant Kumar, Ghanshyam Singh, and Anand Mohan

10.1 Introduction

Recently, the protection of multimedia data from malicious attacks and misuse has become a potential issue. Due to this, the encryption and watermarking are two complementary techniques are being developed to provide protection of multimedia data from illegal copying or misuse of our personal information. However, these two terminologies have their own philosophy, requirement and limitations [1]. Encryption is the commonly used technique to protect multimedia data during the transmission from sender-to-receiver but after decrypted the data at the receiver side, however, the data is similar to the original data and no longer protected. This major limitation of encryption techniques has been addressed in watermarking that protects the multimedia content even after decryption [2]. Watermarking techniques embed imperceptible watermarking information into the main content such that the

A.K. Singh (✉)
Department of Computer Science & Engineering, Jaypee University of Information Technology, Waknaghat, Solan, India
e-mail: amit_245singh@yahoo.com

B. Kumar
Department of Electronics and Communication Engineering, Motilal Nehru National Institute of Technology, Allahabad, India
e-mail: singhbasant@yahoo.com

G. Singh
Department of Electronics and Communication Engineering, Jaypee University of Information Technology, Waknaghat, Solan, India
e-mail: drghanshyam.singh@yahoo.com

A. Mohan
Department of Electronics Engineering, Indian Institute of Technology (BHU), Varanasi, India
e-mail: profanandmohan@gmail.com

© Springer International Publishing AG 2017
A.K. Singh et al. (eds.), *Medical Image Watermarking*, Multimedia Systems and Applications, DOI 10.1007/978-3-319-57699-2_10

watermark is neither removed during normal usage nor causes inconvenience to the users. A watermark can be designed to survive different processes such as decryption, re-encryption, compression and geometrical manipulations [2]. The multimedia documents can be any text, image, audio or a video. Along with the attractive features, the watermarking techniques are also having some issues [2, 3]. The analysis of merits and limitations of these techniques with respect to major watermarking benchmark parameters revealed that it is difficult to achieve satisfactory performance with respect to imperceptibility, robustness, embedding capacity and security, simultaneously [2]. Therefore, it is clear that there are different methods for improving one or a subset of these parameters but they compromise with other remaining parameters.

10.2 Image Watermarking: New Trends and Future Challenges

In this section, we have presented the recent trends and potential research challenges of the state-of-the-art watermarking techniques. It includes watermarking for medical, 3D model watermarking, watermarking in cloud computing and multi-cores environment, biometric watermarking, watermarking using mobile devise and securing online social networks contents. Figure 10.1 show the emerging areas of image watermarking and its related potential issues. Further, the authors have summarized the various techniques in Table 10.1.

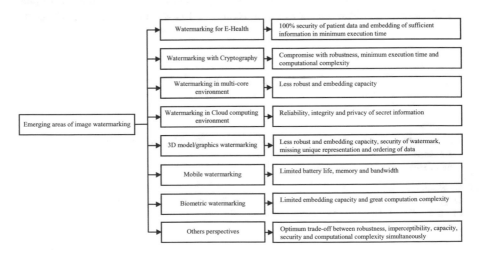

Fig. 10.1 Emerging areas of image watermarking and its related potential issues

Table 10.1 Summary of existing state-of-the-art watermarking techniques

Ref. No.	Proposed objectives	Using techniques to achieved the objectives	Experimental results	Other important considerations
Rocek et al. [23]	Fusion of reversible, zero and RONI watermarking for Medical image	ROI and RONI, Zero watermarking	The average value of PSNR = 81 dB, Average SSIM = 0.999974 Where RONI was 10% of the image size	Test database of 6000 medical images
Thakkar and Srivastava [3]	Robust and secure technique for telemedicine	DWT, SVD, ROI and RONI, Hamming & BCH error correcting code	PSNR >43 dB and WPSNR >52 dB, SSIM is nearly equals to 0.97	Tested for natural, color images and checkmark attacks. Watermark embedding at weight factor = 0.05
Badshah et al. [15]	Lossless compression based medical image watermarking	Lempel-Ziv-Welch (LZW), ROI and LSB	Average compression ratio = 0.054 and PSNR >50 dB	The authors claimed that 100 % accuracy the process of tamper detection and lossless recovery
Nyeem et al. [29]	Medical image watermarking using Content-independent embedding technique	ROI and RONI, LSB	Embedding capacity = 100.40 Kbits, MSSIM >0.999	Set of 370 medical images of different modalities, Image sizes range from 196 × 258 to 600 × 600 (pixels), and image bit-depths are 8-bit and 16-bit
Ma et al. [32]	Reversible data hiding in encrypted images for privacy protection	Image encryption, histogram shift. Boundary map, LSB-planes	10 times larger payloads than other methods. PSNR = 40 dB at embedding rate = 0.4 bpp	Reserving space for embedding before encryption
Zhang et al. [36]	Reversible data hiding technique in encrypted images for privacy protection	AES, Histogram shift	PSNR >55 dB at embedding rate reaches 0.04 bpp, average error pixels = 0. Complexity depends on embedding rate	Under different threshold (T) (1 ≤ T ≤ 8) and secret integers p (q = 10) on 50 images of database
Zheng et al. [37]	Lossless data hiding technique for privacy protection	Chaotic sequence, least significant bits (LSBs), Hamming distance	PSNR of the marked decrypted image is 55.00 dB, embedding rate = 0.041 bit per pixel	Size of all cove image =512 × 512

(continued)

Table 10.1 (continued)

Ref. No.	Proposed objectives	Using techniques to achieved the objectives	Experimental results	Other important considerations
Khor et al. [38]	Parallel watermarking processing in Multicores Environment using medical images	Parallel watermarking processing, multicores technology	The PSNR values are calculated for all images ranging within 48.29 ~ 48.74 dB, Elapsed time = 38.70 s (for parallel) and 738.70 s (sequential) at number of frame = 30 speedup factor = 5.21 ~ 6.60	Parallel modes of watermarking is performed better than sequential mode
Cao et al. [39]	Data hiding technique for higher embedding rate and the image quality	Image encryption, reversible data hiding, sparse coding, K-means singular value decomposition, RC4	PSNR = 40 dB, maximum embedding rate (MER) = 1.01 bits per second.	Complexity = $O(N^2kl)$ + $o(2N^2logN)$, where N = Size of *gray cover image* K = the number of atoms in the dictionary, L = the number of non-zero elements in each coefficient vector. Different databases are considered for experimental purpose. Data extraction and image recovery are separable and reversible. Dictionary training is based on 786 432 patches with size 4 × 4 taken from 48 standard 8-bit grayscale images
Ai et al. [41]	Watermarking technique for 3D triangular mesh models	Feature points, Voronoi patches, DCT	Max PSNR = 88.6837 dB, correlation coefficient >0.6, Max BER = 20% against attacks	Maximum no. of vertex = 362,272, No of patches = 20 is considered for bunny model
Wang et al. [44]	Semi-fragile watermarking technique for the authentication of 3D models	Integral invariants	Robustness against noise increases with the radius of the kernel ball, max BER = 100% at amplitude of noise = 10^{-2}	Bunny model of 34,834 vertices and 69,451 facets using a 24 × 24 monochrome image as the input watermark image

Yang et al. [45]	Steganalytic algorithm for detecting watermark messages embedded in 3D models	Discrete statistic of the histogram of radial coordinates, PCA	Accuracy of up to 99%, Max correlation coefficient = 1.0 at level of noise strength = 0.05%, Number of iteration = 10 and level of quantization = 10	Tested for Bunny, Rabbit, Venus, Dragon and the Horse model. Number of bins = 400
Al-Haj [48]	Blind, imperceptible, and robust watermarking technique to protect the copyright of 3D DIBR images	DWT, SVD, key-based pseudorandom generator	Average SSIM = 0.997, PSNR = 44.14 dB, range of BER is 0 to 0.3 for different attacks, two error probabilities are calculated at BER range from 0.15 to 0.25.	The method is also tested for DIBR-specific attacks
Kejariwal et al. [51]	Watermarking on mobile devices reducing energy consumption	Partitioning scheme, SSL	Reduces the total energy consumed by 80%	Applicable in office environments only
Cao et al. [53]	Preserve the privacy and integrity of digital data on cloud	Logistic-map, chaotic cryptography, histogram shifting algorithm	Max Payload bits (dB) and Payload bpp are 8234 and 0.0314 respectively, MSE = 0	The watermarking technique cannot resist any attacks
Yang et al. [54]	Image watermarking on cloud	SVD, DDWT, Map reduce, Hadoop system	Execution time = 268 min when 1000 images are distributed by the optimization of HPC challenge benchmark	Determine the execution time in two different scenarios
Vatsa et al. [55]	Watermarking for multimodal biometric system for improving robustness, security and accuracy simultaneously	RDWT, Phase congruency model	Verification accuracy = 94%.	Embedding the voice biometric MFC coefficients in a color face image

(continued)

Table 10.1 (continued)

Ref. No.	Proposed objectives	Using techniques to achieved the objectives	Experimental results	Other important considerations
Jain et al. [56]	Security of biometric data using watermarking	Amplitude modulation, steganography, watermarking	Accuracy = 100%	Using fingerprint and face feature vectors as watermark
Wioletta [57]	Biometric watermarking for medical applications	DWT, Hamming distance	Hamming distance is nearly zero	LL component of DWT of image is the most robust against attacks
Bhowmik and Abhayaratne [58]	Scalable blind watermarking for visual contents	Code-stream, bit-plane discarding model, forward discrete wavelet transform, non-uniform quantization based index modulation, Hamming distances	PSNR = 47.43, at Data capacity = 6336 and embedding distortion rate = 84.13	Technique was extended for video watermarking. Robust against scalable media compression
Bhatnagar [1]	High capacity watermarking	Census transform hamming distance, spectral decompositions	Max PSNR = 59.5467 dB and correlation = 0.9994. Max embedding time = 0.9583 s. and min extraction time = 0.4242 s	Free from the false-positive detection problem of singular values
Guo et al. [65]	Progressive Halftone Watermarking for improving the embedding capacity and reliability	Multi-layer halftoning, binary search, Look-Up-Table, naïve Bayes classifier	PSNR = 29.89, Embedding time = 8.4 ms, Correct Decode Rate = 99.32%	Suitable for printing industry
Heidari and Naseri [70]	Quantum watermarking	Quantum representation of digital images , LSB	Max PSNR = 54.1759 dB	Only PSNR performance is determined

10.2.1   *Watermarking for E-health*

The medical image is an important information for identifying disease of the patient. It is also used for insurance claims and evidence in a court of law. Currently, the growth of telemedicine is cause of the increasing the medical images transfer between health-care centers at a distance [4]. Thus, it is needed to ensure that those medical images are unambiguously identified to the correct person and not modified by third party. The digital watermarking is a solution to protect the medical images from unauthorized tampering and modification [2, 3, 5–15]. The digital watermarking techniques compose of watermark embedding and watermark extraction. The objectives of embedding is to insert a message call 'watermark' into a host signal in a secure, imperceptible and inseparable manner. The objective of extraction is to extract the embedded water mark from a watermarked image with the secret key. In recent years, many researchers proposed medical image watermarking for securing of medical information against intentional or accidental alteration/modification to addressing the potential issue in modern radiology. The popular watermarking techniques for the medical application have been reported in [3, 5–22]. In order to that Rocek et al. [23] proposed a fully reversible medical image watermarking by combining the advantages of reversible, zero and RONI watermarking techniques, simultaneously. Initially, the cover image is divided in to region of interest (ROI) and region of non-interest (RONI) parts. The ROI of cover and watermark is combined to generate 'secret share' using Zero watermarking. The 'Secret Share' is embedded as watermark into RONI part of the cover image using Reversible watermarking. Further, the original ROI, RONI and watermark are concatenated to generate a watermarked image. The Peak signal-to-noise ratio (PSNR) and structural similarity index measure (SSIM) performance is experimentally demonstrated and reported that the average value of PSNR and SSIM in images from the test database of 6000 medical images was 81 dB and 0.999974 respectively. In this method, we noticed that the performance (determined by PSNR and SSIM) is RONI dependent. The proposed method was tested with RONI size over 10%. However, another method [24] has a working area with RONI sizes in the range 76–79%, [25] 88–96% and [26] has published results for different types of modalities at RONI size of 88%.

Thakkar and Srivastava [3] proposed a blind medical image watermarking scheme using discrete wavelet transform (DWT) and singular value decomposition (SVD) for telemedicine applications. Initially, the cover image is divided into ROI and RONI parts for embedding the watermarks. DWT is applied on ROI parts of the medical cover image and watermark data in the form of image and text are embedded into the SVD blocks of selected wavelet sub-band of the medical cover. Further, the Hamming and BCH ECC is applying on EPR data and the encoded EPR is embedding into the cover. Moreover, the embedding of watermark bits into selected blocks of the left singular value matrices which do not require any original data in the extraction process to addressing the false positive problem [27], as suffered by SVD based watermarking techniques. The experimental results have shown that the performance of the techniques is good against various kinds of attacks including Checkmark attacks. The method is also found to be robust as compared with other state-of-the-art techniques [13, 28]. However, DWT based watermarking method is suffering from poor directional, phase and shift sensitivity. The computational complexity of the SVD is also high.

A lossless compression based watermarking technique is proposed by Badshah et al. [15] using tele-radiology images. The ROI part of the watermark is considered along with a key to generate a new watermark. The generated watermark is compressed by Lempel–Ziv–Welch (LZW) technique and the compressed watermark is embedding into the RONI part of the cover image. However, the recovered ROI part of watermark is used for tamper detection and lossless recovery. The experimental results established that the performance of the different compression method is investigated and found that the LZW compression technique offer better compression ratio performance than other conventional compression techniques. The method also verifies the tempering in the watermark after extraction and decompression process. Nyeem et al. [29] developed a content-independent watermarking technique using multimodality medical image. The technique computed the RONI part of the cover image and determined the optimum combination of border width and bit-depth for watermark embedding. A set of binary arrays considered as watermark is embedding into the LSB of the RONI part of the cover image. The performance of technique is extensively evaluated in terms of embedding capacity, visual quality of the watermarked image, embedding time and found to be better than other existing technique as proposed by Tsai et al. [30]. However, the method is highly dependent on two defined parameters 'border width' and 'bit-depth'.

10.2.2 Watermarking Using Cryptography

Recently, the medical images play a prominent role for instant diagnosis, understanding of crucial diseases as well as to avoid the misdiagnosis [2, 3] in telemedicine applications. Potential researchers are using fusion of cryptography and watermarking has emerged to disseminate the security to the EPR medical data [6, 9, 31]. However, the main challenge for a good watermarking algorithm is robustness and security against the surviving attacks [6, 9, 31].

Ma et al. [32] proposed a reversible data hiding technique in which the content owner first reserves a sufficient amount space on original image and then the image is encrypted using stream cipher. The performance of the method is compared with other reported techniques [33–35] and found to be better in terms of PSNR and embedding rate. A reversible data hiding technique is also presented by Zhang et al. [36] using advanced encryption standard (AES) encryption. In this technique, a large amount of the cover pixels are estimated before encryption so that extra information is embedded in the estimating errors. The estimating errors and large group of the pixel is encrypted by a special encryption and AES technique respectively. Further, the encrypted estimating errors and the large group of encrypted pixels are concatenated and the final encrypted image is formulated. Experimental results demonstrated that the performance of the proposed method is determined aspect of embedding rate and Peak Signal-to-Noise Ratio (PSNR) and found to be better than other state-of-the art technique [35]. The methods [32, 36] emptied out room before image encryption, and achieved excellent performance. Unfortunately, the operating of image encryption and data embedding is inseparable, which can not satisfy the application requirement of privacy protection, as reported by Zheng et al. [37]. Zheng et al. [37] proposed a reversible data hiding technique using a chaotic sequence for encrypting original image. In the embedding process of secret data, the least significant bits (LSB) of the encrypted original bits are compressed and reserve some space for additional data using Hamming distance. Experimental results demonstrated that the method performed better than other reported techniques [33–35] in term of embedding rate and the quality of marked decrypted images.

Khor et al. [38] have developed two different mode of watermarking process in the form sequential and parallel for medical application. In the parallel watermarking process, generated frames of ultrasound images were loaded into a quad core microprocessor and create a job on the scheduler. The job is then divided into tasks according to the number of cores is available in the microprocessor. Upon the task is completed, all the frames are concatenated into an array and submit back to the microprocessor. The concatenate output result retrieved from the microprocessor is writing into a digital imaging and communications in medicine (DICOM) file. Finally, the job is deleted under the selected circumstances. An experiment result demonstrated that the elapsed time for watermarking embedding process on sequential watermarking processing is greater than that of the parallel watermarking processing. In addition to that the efficiency of parallel watermarking processing is much faster than that of the sequential process at complete tampered watermarked. Cao et al. [39] presented a reversible data hiding technique using patch-level sparse coding. In the embedding process of watermark, the cover image is divided into different patches and the selected patches are represented by sparse coefficients, and the corresponding remaining errors are encoded and reversibly embedded into the other non-selected patches using standard reversible data hiding algorithm. Finally, the room preserved and self-embedded image is encrypted to generate the encrypted cover image. Furthermore, the secret data and learned dictionary is embedded into the encrypted image. The experimental results demonstrated that the embedding rate and image quality is better than other reported techniques.

10.2.3 3D Model/Graphics Watermarking

Currently, 3D model/graphics are widely used in medical imaging, industrial, multimedia, entertainment, virtual reality, video games, Web3D, MPEG4 and computer aided design [40, 41]. However, the copyright protection and authentication problems have become a potential issues arising with their increasing demand/use [41]. Digital watermarking of 3D objects/model, as reported by some researcher has been considered an efficient tool for solving these increasing problems.

In the early stage, Ohbuchi et al. [42, 43] proposed different 3D object models such as triangle similarity quadruple (TSQ) embedding algorithm, tetrahedral volume ratio (TVR) embedding algorithm, triangle strip peeling symbol sequence (TSPS) embedding algorithm, polygon stencil pattern (PSP) embedding algorithm, etc. and examined that the presented models are not sufficient robust against attacks of mesh simplification and re-meshing [41]. Ai et al. [41] proposed an watermarking technique for 3D triangular mesh models using feature points as detected from selected area the model. The watermark information is repeatedly embedding into the corresponding range image of each Voronoi patch. The method is imperceptible and highly robust for mesh simplification noise amplitude, cropping and combination of simplification and cropping attacks. In addition to that the authors are compared some state of the art 3D watermarking techniques in terms of embedding capacity, the methods are blind or non-blind and attacks resistant in tabular format. Wang et al. [44] proposed a semi-fragile watermarking algorithm for authentication of 3D model based on integral invariants using spatial domain technique. The transformed image watermark information by Arnold is embedding into the mesh. The method is robust against additive noise.

Yang et al. [45] proposed a steganalytic algorithm for embedding watermarks based on discrete static of histogram of radical coordinates by two different 3D watermarking as presented in [46, 47]. The experimental results have been shown that the method is robust and better embedding distortion than two other state of the art watermarking algorithms [46, 47] against attacks. Al-Haj [48] proposed a robust 3D depth-image-based rendering (DIBR) digital image watermarking algorithm using fusion of DWT and the SVD for 3D applications. Initially, DWT is applied on random sub-image generated from the original image using chaos-based approach. The selected sub-bands of the DWT are divided into different sub-blocks. Further, SVD is applied on each sub-block. The random sequence watermark bits are now embedded into the suitable blocks of the random sub-image. The simulation results have been shown that the algorithm is imperceptible, and robust against attacks including DIBR-specific attacks. The robustness performance in terms of BER of the proposed algorithm is compared with other state-of-the-art watermarking techniques [49, 50]. Moreover, two error probabilities in terms of false alarm and false rejection are also determined and found that these probabilities are highly depends on length of the watermark.

10.2.4 Watermarking for Mobile Devise

Generally, the robust and secure wavelet based watermarking techniques are computationally expensive and adds to the drain of available energy in mobile devices.

The energy characterization of state-of-the-art wavelet based image watermarking techniques has been discussed by Kejariwal et al. [51] and proposed two proxy-based partitioning techniques for energy efficient watermarking on mobile/tablet devices. These techniques is divided the watermarking tasks between a proxy server and the mobile device. Further, the method also studied the impact of security and visual quality of image on energy consumption. The techniques is tried to balance between reducing energy and secure the multimedia data.

10.2.5   Watermarking in Cloud Computing Environments

With the development of cloud computing, various applications are using cloud storage services to manage digital data remotely via internet [52]. In order to that some researcher proposed watermarking techniques to enhance the security of the digital data in cloud computing platforms.

Cao et al. [53] discussed a techniques using combination of watermarking and encryption in cloud computing environment. Initially, the method encrypted the original image using Logistic map-based chaotic encryption algorithm and divide the encrypted image into the number of blocks. The watermark information is embedding into the selected blocks of the encrypted image using histogram shifting algorithm. The cloud service providers stored the encrypted image containing the embedded watermark information on cloud. However, the proposed method was using fragile watermark algorithm which cannot resist any attacks. Yang et al. [54] proposed a watermarking method in Hadoop computing environments using fusion of singular value decomposition (SVD) and distributed discrete wavelet transformation (DDWT). The Eigen value of the cover image is modified with Eigen value of the watermark image. The modified image is then embedding into the third level of DDWT. The simulation results demonstrated that the execution time is reduced when the '1000' of images distributed with high performance computer instead of the images distributed evenly.

10.2.6   Biometric Watermarking

The biometric authentication systems have inherent advantage over traditional personal identification techniques [55]. However, the security and integrity of biometric data has become a potential issue [56]. Researchers are securing biometric data by suitable watermarking techniques [55, 56].

Vatsa et al. [55] proposed a biometric watermarking method in which biometric voice template is embedding into the color face image of the same individual using redundant discrete wavelet transformation (RDWT). The experimental results have been shown that the accuracy of the RDWT watermarking method is better than the DWT watermarking and the method robust for different kind of attacks. Further, the statistical evaluation is performed on the multi-biometrics algorithm and found to be robust to different kinds of attacks. Jain et al. [56] introduced biometric data hiding technique in two different application scenarios. In the first scenario, the cover image is not related to the hidden data in any way. The actual fingerprint minutiae information of 85 bytes is embedded into the cover synthetic fingerprint image. Further, the security of the cover image carrying biometric information is enhanced by the encryption techniques. In second scenario, the 14 eigen-face coefficients of 56 bytes instead of minutiae are embedding into the fingerprint image. The experimental results have shown that the 100% accuracy has been achieved from all of the 640 watermarked images. Wioletta [57] proposed another biometric watermarking algorithm using DWT in which iris code is considered as watermark. The medical cover gray image is decomposed by the DWT and the biometric watermark is embedding into the selected top left corner of each sub-band of DWT cover. The performance of proposed algorithm is determined against three important attacks by Hamming distance between embedded and extracted iris code in the cover medical image.

10.2.7   Other Perspectives

In recent image and video coding techniques, the scalable coding has become a genuine functionality in which scalable coders generate scalable bit streams demonstrating content in hierarchical layers of increasing audiovisual quality and increasing spatiotemporal resolutions [58]. However, the watermarking for scalable coded information is more challenging than that of the traditional watermarking techniques [59–62].

In this application scenarios, Bhowmik and Abhayaratne [58] developed a robust and blind scalable watermarking technique based on bit-plane discarding model in which hierarchical embedded code-stream is generated. Further, the generated code-stream is then truncated at various embedding distortion rate to create watermarked images. The extraction and authentication is performed using a blind extractor. The algorithm is developed based on the bit-plane discarding model used in scalable content adaptation. The experimental results demonstrated that the concept was verified for image and video sequences. The performance of the method is extensively evaluated in terms of embedding distortion rate and compression ratio. The method is robust against scalable content adaptation attacks. Further, the data capacity performance the method is better than other non-scalable based reported techniques [59, 63, 64]. Moreover, the robustness performance of the proposed method was determined for video watermarking.

A robust and high capacity watermarking technique is presented in [1] using fusion of Census and SVD transform domain techniques. Initially, the census transform is applied on each pixel of the cover image and is mapped in to the bit string. The minimum Hamming distance is calculated between key and bit string of the pixel for embedding purpose. Further, the spectral decomposition is applied on the sequence of selected pixels and the watermark is embedded in the spectral coefficients. The performance of different spectral decompositions are determined and found that the robustness performance of Hankel spectral decomposition (HSD) is better than that of the Circulant and Topelitz spectral decomposition. The simulation results have demonstrated that the method is robust and high capacity at acceptable visual quality of the watermarked image. The method also addressing the false detection problem as suffered by SVD based watermarking. The complexity of the method is also impressive.

Guo et al. [65] presents a halftoning-based multilayer watermarking technique with low computational complexity. The method is using noise-balanced error diffusion to achieved high embedding capacity and improved security aspect. Binary search and Look-Up-Table (LUT) method are using for embedding the multiple watermarks. However, Least-Mean-Square (LMS) and naïve Bayes classifier are using to extract the embedded watermarks information. The authors are reported that the suggested method is embedding multiple watermarks in 8.4 ms and 2MB is required to store the proposed compressed reference table. The performance of the method in terms of correct decode rate (CDR) and Human visual system Peak Signal-to- Noise Ratio (HPSNR), and efficiency (complexity and processing time) is better than other reported techniques [66–69]. Heidari and Naseri [70] proposed a quantum watermarking method in which quantum signal/information is embedding into the quantum cover image. In this method, the scrambled watermark information along with the keys are embedding into the cover using LSB technique. The performance is validated in terms of PSNR and authors reported that the method is robust. Further, simulation results is demonstrated that PSNR performance is improved 6% than other reported technique as proposed by Jiang et al. [71].

10.3   Research Challenges in Existing State-of-the-Art Watermarking Techniques

The foregoing section presented a comprehensive survey of various state-of-the-art image watermarking techniques. We have noticed that numerous robust and secure watermarking algorithms have been proposed but there has been rat race situation between robustness of watermark and malicious attacks; making robust watermarking an interesting challenging area for researchers. The potential challenges have also been discussed in Chap. 2, however, important investigations from the various reported watermarking techniques are summarized as follows.

– Various watermarking techniques have been reported by noted researchers for telemedicine applications [2, 3, 5–26, 28–30]. However, it is clear that there are different methods for improving one or a subset of the benchmark parameters such as robustness, capacity, imperceptibility, security and complexity but they compromise with other remaining parameters. Embedding of sufficient information in cover media with minimum execution time is a challenging/crucial task for practical applications. We have noticed that 100% security of cover and watermark(s) information is a challenging issue. With the best of authors knowledge no method are providing the optimal trade-off between these benchmark parameters simultaneously for telemedicine application.
– A group of researchers are focused on the watermark security using fusion of cryptography and watermarking [6, 9, 32–39]. For the security issues, encrypting watermark information before watermarking has become unavoidable, but the delay encountered during the embedding and extraction of watermark is also an important factor in real-time applications [8]. Therefore, the watermark constitution by using encryption techniques should be simple to save execution time. For the tele-diagnosis, the speed has become an important factor if the situation

demands [8, 10, 11]. We have also noticed that the security and embedding capacity of the watermark information is enhanced; however the researchers are compromising with other important parameters such as robustness, complexity and execution time.

- The watermarking techniques for 3D objects are reported by noted researcher in [40–50]. However, 3D model based watermarking techniques are suffering from less data embedding capacity and robust, no any unique representation exists and implicit ordering of data, and easily destroy the watermark embedded into the model [41] and selection of a suitable feature space, in which the watermark information is inserted [44].
- The watermarking technique [51] for mobile devices has been proposed. However, the mobile devices have limited battery life due to amount of computational load placed by applications, memory and bandwidth. The digital watermarking tasks place an extra burden on the available energy in these devices [51]. Further, the security of the watermark(s) and is also a potential issue.
- Several researchers proposed watermarking techniques in cloud computing environments [52–54]. However, the reliability integrity and privacy of multimedia information stored remotely has become a potential challenge [52–54].
- Biometric watermarking techniques [55–57] enhanced the security of biometric template(s)/watermark(s) information. However, the biometric watermarking has limited embedding capacity and large computation complexity.
- Scalable watermarking technique for visual contents has been proposed in [58]. However, the watermarking for scalable coded content is far more challenging than that of the traditional watermarking techniques [59–62].
- Multilayer watermarking technique is presented in [65] with low computational complexity. However, the processing efficiency for large size of multimedia data is a potential issue in practical applications.
- In [70, 71], the quantum watermarking techniques are presented. However, the robustness performance under different attacks is required to enhance at low computational complexity.

10.4 Summary

Novel/improved watermarking techniques are invented regularly. Some of the watermarking techniques are intended for specific applications, while the others are not well recognized yet but have a great potential. This chapter has given a state-of-the-art overview of different watermarking techniques in various applications environments. The chapter also discussed potential challenges that the watermarking process face. Further, the chapter presented the brief summary of the different techniques has been tabulated.

References

1. G. Bhatnagar, Robust covert communication using high capacity watermarking. Multimedia Tools Appl. **76**, 3783 (2016). doi:10.1007/s11042-016-3978-x
2. A.K. Singh, Some new techniques of improved wavelet domain watermarking for medical images, Ph.D. Thesis, Department of Computer Engineering, NIT Kurukshetra, India, 2015
3. F.N. Thakkar, V.K. Srivastava, A blind medical image watermarking: DWT-SVD based robust and secure approach for telemedicine applications. Multimedia Tools Appl. **76**(3), 3669–3697 (2016)
4. World Health Organization, Telemedicine opportunities and developments, Report on the second global survey on eHealth, 2010
5. A. Zear, A.K. Singh, P. Kumar, Multiple watermarking for healthcare applications. J. Intell. Syst. (2016). doi:10.1515/jisys-2016-0036
6. A. Sharma, A.K. Singh, S.P. Ghrera, Robust and secure multiple watermarking technique for medical images. Wirel. Pers. Commun. **92**(4), 1611–1624 (2017)
7. A. Zear, A.K. Singh, P. Kumar, A proposed secure multiple watermarking technique based on DWT, DCT and SVD for application in medicine. Multimedia Tools Appl. (2016). doi:10.1007/s11042-016-3862-8
8. A.K. Singh, Improved hybrid technique for robust and imperceptible multiple watermarking using medical images. Multimedia Tools Appl. **76**(6), 8881–8900 (2017)
9. R. Pandey, A.K. Singh, B. Kumar, A. Mohan, Iris based secure NROI multiple eye image watermarking for teleophthalmology. Multimedia Tools Appl. **75**(22), 14381–14397 (2016)
10. A.K. Singh, M. Dave, A. Mohan, Hybrid technique for robust and imperceptible multiple watermarking using medical images. J. Multimedia Tools Appl. **75**(14), 8381–8401 (2015)
11. A.K. Singh, M. Dave, A. Mohan, Multilevel encrypted text watermarking on medical images using spread-spectrum in DWT domain. Wirel. Pers. Commun. **83**(3), 2133–2150 (2015)
12. A.K. Singh, M. Dave, A. Mohan, Robust and secure multiple watermarking in wavelet domain, a special issue on advanced signal processing technologies and systems for healthcare applications (ASPTSHA). J. Med. Imaging Health Inf. **5**(2), 406–414 (2015)
13. A.K. Singh, B. Kumar, M. Dave, A. Mohan, Multiple watermarking on medical images using selective DWT coefficients. J. Med. Imaging Health Inf. **5**(3), 607–614 (2015)
14. A.K. Singh, B. Kumar, M. Dave, A. Mohan, Robust and imperceptible spread-spectrum watermarking for telemedicine applications. Proc. Natl. Acad. Sci., India Sect. A: Phys. Sci. **85**(2), 295–301 (2015)
15. G. Badshah, S.-C. Liew, J.M. Zain, M. Ali, Watermark compression in medical image watermarking using lempel-ziv-welch (LZW) lossless compression technique. J. Digit. Imaging **29**(2), 216–225 (2016)
16. F. Rahimi, H. Rabbani, A dual adaptive watermarking scheme in contourlet domain for DICOM images. Biomed. Eng. Online **10**, 53 (2011). doi:10.1186/1475-925X-10-53
17. O.M. Al-Qershi, B.E. Khoo, Authentication and data hiding using a hybridROI-based watermarking scheme for DICOM images. J. Digit. Imaging **24**(21), 114–125 (2011)
18. C.K. Tan, J.C. Ng, X. Xu, C.L. Poh, Y.L. Guan, K. Sheah, Security protection of DICOM medical images using dual-layer reversible watermarking with tamper detection capability. J. Digit. Imaging **24**(3), 528–540 (2011)
19. H. Rahmani, R. Mortezaei, M.E. Moghaddam, A new lossless watermarking scheme based on DCT coefficients, in 6th International Conference on Digital Content, Multimedia Technology and its Applications, Seoul, Korea (South), pp. 28–33, ISBN: 978-1-4244-7607-7, 2010
20. H.H. Tsai, H.C. Tseng, Y.S. Lai, Robust lossless image watermarking based on α-trimmed mean algorithm and support vector machine. J. Syst. Softw. **83**(6), 1015–1028 (2010)
21. W. Pan, G. Coatrieux, J. Montagner, N. Cuppens, F. Cuppens, Ch. Roux, Comparison of some reversible watermarking methods in application to medical images, in 31st Annual International Conference of the IEEE EMBS, Minneapolis, Minnesota, USA, 2–6 Sept 2009, pp. 2172–2175

22. I.F. Kallel, M.S. Bouhlel, J.C. Lapayre, Improved Tian's method for medical image reversible watermarking. GVIP J. **7**(2), 1–5 (2007)
23. A. Rocek, K. Slavicek, O. Dostal, M. Javornik, A new approach to fully-reversible watermarking in medical imagingwith breakthrough visibility. Biomed. Signal Process. Control **29**, 44–52 (2016)
24. J. Mašek, R. Burget, J. Karásek, V. Uher, S. Güney, Evolutionary improved object detector for ultrasound images, in 36th International Conference on Telecommunications and Signal processing Rome, Italy, pp. 586–590, 2013
25. R. Eswaraiah, E.S. Reddy, Robust medical image watermarking technique foraccurate detection of tampers inside region of interest and recovering original region of interest. IET Image Process. **9**(8), 615–625 (2015)
26. O.M. Al-Qershi, B.E. Khoo, ROI–based tamper detection and recovery for medical images using reversible watermarking technique, in IEEE International Conference on Information Theory and Information Security, Beijing, pp. 151–155, 2010
27. X.-P. Zhang, K. Li, Comments on "SVD-based watermarking scheme for protecting rightful ownership". IEEE Trans. Multimedia **7**(2), 593–594 (2005)
28. S.A. Parah, J.A. Sheikh, F. Ahad, N.A. Loan, G.M. Bhat, Information hiding in medical images: a robust medical image watermarking system for E-healthcare. Multimedia Tools Appl. **76**(8), 10599–10633 (2017)
29. H. Nyeem, W. Boles, C. Boyd, Content-independent embedding scheme for multi-modal medical image watermarking. Biomed. Eng. Online **14**, 7 (2015). doi:10.1186/1475-925X-14-7
30. P. Tsai, Y.C. Hu, H.L. Yeh, Reversible image hiding scheme using predictive coding and histogram shifting. Sig. Process. **89**(6), 1129–1143 (2009)
31. S.M. Mousavi, A. Naghsh, S.A.R. Abu-Bakar, Watermarking techniques used in medical images: A survey. J. Digit. Imaging **27**(6), 714–729 (2014)
32. K. Ma, W. Zhang, X. Zhao, N. Yu, F. Li, Reversible data hiding in encrypted images by reserving room before encryption. IEEE Trans. Inf. Forensics Secur. **8**(3), 553–562 (2013)
33. X. Zhang, Reversible data hiding in encrypted images. IEEE Signal Process. Lett. **18**(4), 255–258 (2011)
34. W. Hong, T. Chen, H. Wu, An improved reversible data hiding in encrypted images using side match. IEEE Signal Process. Lett. **19**(4), 199–202 (2012)
35. X. Zhang, Separable reversible data hiding in encrypted image. IEEE Trans. Inf. Forensics Security **7**(2), 826–832 (2012)
36. W. Zhang, K. Ma, N. Yu, Reversibility improved data hiding in encrypted images. Signal Process. **94**, 118–127 (2014)
37. S. Zheng, D. Li, D. Hu, D. Ye, J.W. LinaWang, Lossless data hiding for encrypted images with high capacity. Multimedia Tools Appl. **75**(21), 13765–13778 (2016)
38. H.L. Khor, S.-C. Liew, J.M. Zain, Parallel digital watermarking process on ultrasound medical images in multicores environment. Int. J. Biomed. Imaging **2016**, 1–14 (2016)
39. X. Cao, D. Ling, X. Wei, D. Meng, X. Guo, High capacity reversible data hiding in encrypted images by patch-level sparse representation. IEEE Trans. Cybernet. **46**(5), 1132–1143 (2016)
40. M.-W. Chao, C.-h. Lin, Y. Cheng-Wei, T.-Y. Lee, A high capacity 3D steganography algorithm. IEEE Trans. Vis. Comput. Graph. **15**(2), 274–284 (2009)
41. Q.S. Ai, Q. Liu, Z.D. Zhou, L. Yang, S.Q. Xie, A new digital watermarking scheme for 3D triangular mesh models. Signal Process. **89**(11), 2159–2170 (2009)
42. R. Ohbuchi, H. Masuda, M. Aono, Data embedding algorithms for geometrical and non-geometrical targets in three-dimensional polygonal models. Comput. Commun. **21**(15), 1344–1354 (1998)
43. R. Ohbuchi, S. Takahashi, T. Miyazawa, A. Mukaiyama, Watermarking 3D polygonal meshes in the mesh spectral domain, in Proceedings of Graphics Interface, San Francisco, 7–9 June 2001, pp. 9–17
44. Y.-P. Wang, H. Shi-Min, A new watermarking method for 3D models based on integral invariants. IEEE Trans. Vis. Comput. Graph. **15**(2), 285–294 (2009)

45. Y. Yang, R. Pintus, H. Rushmeier, I. Ivrissimtzis, A 3D steganalytic algorithm and steganalysis-resistant watermarking. IEEE Trans. Vis. Comput. Graph. **23**(2), 1002–1013 (2017)
46. Y Yang, R. Pintus, H. Rushmeier, I. Ivrissimtzis, A steganalytic algorithm for 3D polygonal meshes, in IEEE International Conference on Image Processing (ICIP), Paris, France, Oct 2014, pp. 4782–4786
47. J.-W. Cho, R. Prost, H.-Y. Jung, An oblivious watermarking for 3-D polygonal meshes using distribution of vertex norms. IEEE Trans. Signal Process. **55**(1), 142–155 (2007)
48. A. Al-Haj, M.E. Farfoura, A. Mohammad, Transform-based watermarking of 3D depth-image-based-rendering images. Measurement **95**, 405–417 (2017)
49. Y.H. Lin, J.L. Wu, A digital blind watermarking for depth-image based rendering 3D images. IEEE Trans. Broadcasting **57**(2), 602–611 (2011)
50. H.D. Kim, J.W. Lee, T.W. Oh, H.K. Lee, Robust DT-CWT Watermarking for DIBR 3D Images. IEEE Trans. Broadcasting **58**(4), 533–543 (2012)
51. A. Kejariwal, S. Gupta, A. Nicolau, N.D. Dutt, R. Gupta, Energy efficient watermarking on mobile devices using proxy-based partitioning. IEEE Trans. VLSI Syst. **14**(6), 625–636 (2006)
52. S.G. Shini, T. Tony, K. Chithraranja, Cloud based medical image exchange-security challenges. Process. Eng. **38**, 3454–3461 (2012)
53. X. Cao, F. Zhangjie, X. Sun, A privacy-preserving outsourcing data storage scheme with fragile digital watermarking-based data auditing. J. Elect. Computer Eng. **2016**, 1–7 (2016)
54. C.-T. Yang, C.-H. Lin, G.-L. Chang, Implementation of image watermarking processes on cloud computing environments, security-enriched urban computing and smart grid. Ser. Commun. Computer Inf. Sci. **223**, 131–140 (2011)
55. M. Vatsa, R. Singh, A. Noore, Feature based RDWT watermarking for multimodal biometric system. Image Vis. Comput. **27**(3), 293–304 (2009)
56. A.K. Jain, U. Uludag, Hiding biometric data. IEEE Trans. Pattern Anal. Mach. Intell. **25**(11), 1494–1498 (2003)
57. WIOLETTA, Biometric watermarking for medical images–example of IRIS code. Tech. Trans., 409–416 (2013)
58. D. Bhowmik, C. Abhayaratne, Quality scalability aware watermarking for visual content. IEEE Trans. Image Process. **25**(11), 5158–5172 (2016)
59. F. Huo, X. Gao, A wavelet based image watermarking scheme, in *Proceedings 2006 IEEE International Conference on Image Processing*, Atlanta, Georgia, USA, 2006, pp. 2573–2576
60. A.V. Subramanyam, S. Emmanuel, Partially compressed-encrypted domain robust JPEG image watermarking. Multimedia Tools Appl. **71**(3), 1311–1331 (2014)
61. H.-T. Hu, L.-Y. Hsu, Exploring DWT–SVD–DCT feature parameters for robust multiple watermarking against JPEG and JPEG2000 compression. Comput. Electr. Eng. **41**, 52–63 (2015)
62. N. Cai, N. Zhu, S. Weng, B.W.-K. Ling, Difference angle quantization index modulation scheme for image watermarking. Signal Process. Image Commun. **34**, 52–60 (2015)
63. L. Xie, G.R. Arce, Joint wavelet compression and authentication watermarking. Proc. Int. Conf. Image Process. **2**, 427–431 (1998)
64. P. Meerwald, Quantization watermarking in the JPEG2000 coding pipeline, in *Communications and Multimedia Security Issues of the New Century*, vol. 64 of the series IFIP, The International Federation for Information Processing, 2001, pp. 69–79
65. J.M. Guo, G.-H. Lai, K. Wong, C.C. Li, Progressive Halftone watermarking using multilayer table lookup strategy. IEEE Trans. Image Process. **24**(7), 2009–2024 (2015)
66. C.C.S. JM Guo, Y.F. Liu, H. Lee, J.D. Lee, Oriented modulation for watermarking in direct binary search halftone images. IEEE Trans. Image Process. **21**(9), 4117–4127 (2012)
67. S.C. Pei, J.M. Guo, H. Lee, Novel robust watermarking technique in dithering halftone images. IEEE Signal Process. Lett. **12**(4), 333–336 (2005)
68. J.M. Guo, Y.F. Liu, Hiding multitone watermarks in halftone images. IEEE Multimedia **17**(1), 34–43 (2010)

69. J.M. Guo, Y.F. Liu, Halftone-image security improving using overall minimal-error searching. IEEE Trans. Image Process. **20**(10), 2800–2812 (2011)
70. S. Heidari, M. Naseri, A novel LSB based quantum watermarking. Int. J. Theor. Phys. **55**(10), 4205–4218 (2016)
71. N. Jiang, N. Zhao, L. Wang, LSB based quantum image steganography algorithm. Int. J. Theor. Phys. **55**(1), 107–123 (2016)

Printed in the United States
By Bookmasters